# 50% OFF Online CPHQ Prep Course!

Dear Customer,

We consider it an honor and a privilege that you chose our CPHQ Study Guide. As a way of showing our appreciation and to help us better serve you, we have partnered with Mometrix Test Preparation to offer **50% off their online CPHQ Prep Course**. Many CPHQ courses are needlessly expensive and don't deliver enough value. With their course, you get access to the best CPHQ prep material, and you only pay half price.

**Mometrix has structured their online course to perfectly complement your printed study guide**. The CPHQ Prep Course contains **in-depth lessons** that cover all the most important topics, **over 700 practice questions** to ensure you feel prepared, and **over 350 digital flashcards**, so you can study while you're on the go.

**Online CPHQ Prep Course**

***Topics Include:***

- Organizational Leadership
  - Structure and Integration
  - Regulatory, Accreditation, and External Recognition
  - Education, Training, and Communication
- Health Data Analytics
  - Epidemiological Theory and Surveillance
  - Data Management Systems and Data Display
- Performance and Process Improvement
  - Evaluation of Team Performance
  - Performance Improvement Plan Development
- Patient Safety
  - Culture of Safety
  - Risk Management

***Course Features:***

- CPHQ Study Guide
  - Get content that complements our best-selling study guide.
- Full-Length Practice Tests
  - With over 700 practice questions, you can test yourself again and again.
- Mobile Friendly
  - If you need to study on the go, the course is easily accessible from your mobile device.
- CPHQ Flashcards
  - Their course includes a flashcard mode consisting of over 350 content cards to help you study.

To receive this discount, visit their website: mometrix.com/university/cphq or simply scan this QR code with your smartphone. At the checkout page, enter the discount code: **TPBCPHQ50**

If you have any questions or concerns, please don't hesitate to contact them at universityhelp@mometrix.com.

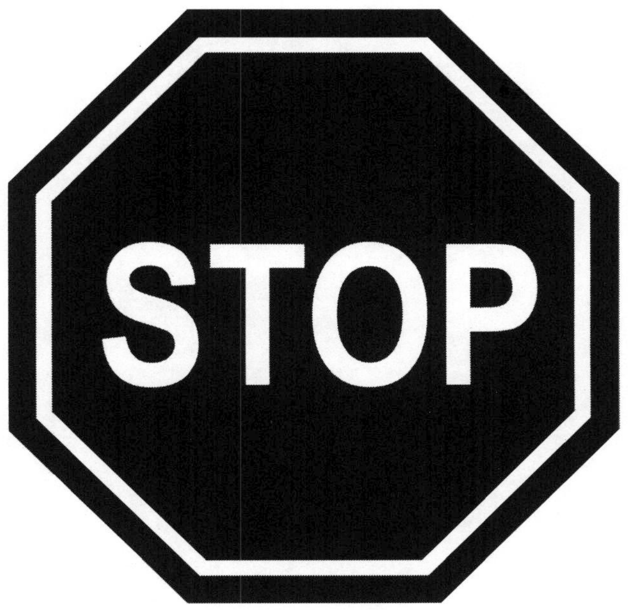


# FREE Test Taking Tips Video/DVD Offer

To better serve you, we created videos covering test taking tips that we want to give you for FREE. **These videos cover world-class tips that will help you succeed on your test.**

We just ask that you send us feedback about this product. Please let us know what you thought about it—whether good, bad, or indifferent.

To get your **FREE videos**, you can use the QR code below or email freevideos@studyguideteam.com with "Free Videos" in the subject line and the following information in the body of the email:

a. The title of your product

b. Your product rating on a scale of 1-5, with 5 being the highest

c. Your feedback about the product

If you have any questions or concerns, please don't hesitate to contact us at info@studyguideteam.com.

Thank you!

# CPHQ Prep 2023-2024

## 3 Practice Tests and Study Guide for the NAHQ Certified Professional in Healthcare Quality Exam [4th Edition]

Joshua Rueda

Written and edited by TPB Publishing.



ISBN 13: 9781637759295
ISBN 10: 1637759290

# Table of Contents

# Quick Overview

As you draw closer to taking your exam, effective preparation becomes more and more important. Thankfully, you have this study guide to help you get ready. Use this guide to help keep your studying on track and refer to it often.

This study guide contains several key sections that will help you be successful on your exam. The guide contains tips for what you should do the night before and the day of the test. Also included are test-taking tips. Knowing the right information is not always enough. Many well-prepared test takers struggle with exams. These tips will help equip you to accurately read, assess, and answer test questions.

A large part of the guide is devoted to showing you what content to expect on the exam and to helping you better understand that content. In this guide are practice test questions so that you can see how well you have grasped the content. Then, answer explanations are provided so that you can understand why you missed certain questions.

Don't try to cram the night before you take your exam. This is not a wise strategy for a few reasons. First, your retention of the information will be low. Your time would be better used by reviewing information you already know rather than trying to learn a lot of new information. Second, you will likely become stressed as you try to gain a large amount of knowledge in a short amount of time. Third, you will be depriving yourself of sleep. So be sure to go to bed at a reasonable time the night before. Being well-rested helps you focus and remain calm.

Be sure to eat a substantial breakfast the morning of the exam. If you are taking the exam in the afternoon, be sure to have a good lunch as well. Being hungry is distracting and can make it difficult to focus. You have hopefully spent lots of time preparing for the exam. Don't let an empty stomach get in the way of success!

When travelling to the testing center, leave earlier than needed. That way, you have a buffer in case you experience any delays. This will help you remain calm and will keep you from missing your appointment time at the testing center.

Be sure to pace yourself during the exam. Don't try to rush through the exam. There is no need to risk performing poorly on the exam just so you can leave the testing center early. Allow yourself to use all of the allotted time if needed.

Remain positive while taking the exam even if you feel like you are performing poorly. Thinking about the content you should have mastered will not help you perform better on the exam.

Once the exam is complete, take some time to relax. Even if you feel that you need to take the exam again, you will be well served by some down time before you begin studying again. It's often easier to convince yourself to study if you know that it will come with a reward!

# Test-Taking Strategies

## 1. Predicting the Answer

When you feel confident in your preparation for a multiple-choice test, try predicting the answer before reading the answer choices. This is especially useful on questions that test objective factual knowledge. By predicting the answer before reading the available choices, you eliminate the possibility that you will be distracted or led astray by an incorrect answer choice. You will feel more confident in your selection if you read the question, predict the answer, and then find your prediction among the answer choices. After using this strategy, be sure to still read all of the answer choices carefully and completely. If you feel unprepared, you should not attempt to predict the answers. This would be a waste of time and an opportunity for your mind to wander in the wrong direction.

## 2. Reading the Whole Question

Too often, test takers scan a multiple-choice question, recognize a few familiar words, and immediately jump to the answer choices. Test authors are aware of this common impatience, and they will sometimes prey upon it. For instance, a test author might subtly turn the question into a negative, or he or she might redirect the focus of the question right at the end. The only way to avoid falling into these traps is to read the entirety of the question carefully before reading the answer choices.

## 3. Looking for Wrong Answers

Long and complicated multiple-choice questions can be intimidating. One way to simplify a difficult multiple-choice question is to eliminate all of the answer choices that are clearly wrong. In most sets of answers, there will be at least one selection that can be dismissed right away. If the test is administered on paper, the test taker could draw a line through it to indicate that it may be ignored; otherwise, the test taker will have to perform this operation mentally or on scratch paper. In either case, once the obviously incorrect answers have been eliminated, the remaining choices may be considered. Sometimes identifying the clearly wrong answers will give the test taker some information about the correct answer. For instance, if one of the remaining answer choices is a direct opposite of one of the eliminated answer choices, it may well be the correct answer. The opposite of obviously wrong is obviously right! Of course, this is not always the case. Some answers are obviously incorrect simply because they are irrelevant to the question being asked. Still, identifying and eliminating some incorrect answer choices is a good way to simplify a multiple-choice question.

## 4. Don't Overanalyze

Anxious test takers often overanalyze questions. When you are nervous, your brain will often run wild, causing you to make associations and discover clues that don't actually exist. If you feel that this may be a problem for you, do whatever you can to slow down during the test. Try taking a deep breath or counting to ten. As you read and consider the question, restrict yourself to the particular words used by the author. Avoid thought tangents about what the author *really* meant, or what he or she was *trying* to say. The only things that matter on a multiple-choice test are the words that are actually in the question. You must avoid reading too much into a multiple-choice question, or supposing that the writer meant something other than what he or she wrote.

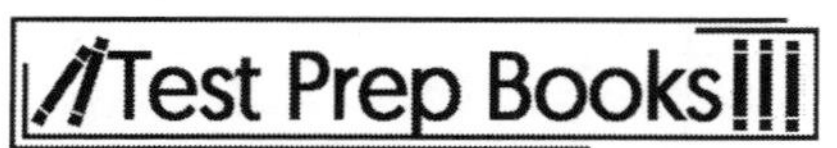

## 5. No Need for Panic

It is wise to learn as many strategies as possible before taking a multiple-choice test, but it is likely that you will come across a few questions for which you simply don't know the answer. In this situation, avoid panicking. Because most multiple-choice tests include dozens of questions, the relative value of a single wrong answer is small. As much as possible, you should compartmentalize each question on a multiple-choice test. In other words, you should not allow your feelings about one question to affect your success on the others. When you find a question that you either don't understand or don't know how to answer, just take a deep breath and do your best. Read the entire question slowly and carefully. Try rephrasing the question a couple of different ways. Then, read all of the answer choices carefully. After eliminating obviously wrong answers, make a selection and move on to the next question.

## 6. Confusing Answer Choices

When working on a difficult multiple-choice question, there may be a tendency to focus on the answer choices that are the easiest to understand. Many people, whether consciously or not, gravitate to the answer choices that require the least concentration, knowledge, and memory. This is a mistake. When you come across an answer choice that is confusing, you should give it extra attention. A question might be confusing because you do not know the subject matter to which it refers. If this is the case, don't eliminate the answer before you have affirmatively settled on another. When you come across an answer choice of this type, set it aside as you look at the remaining choices. If you can confidently assert that one of the other choices is correct, you can leave the confusing answer aside. Otherwise, you will need to take a moment to try to better understand the confusing answer choice. Rephrasing is one way to tease out the sense of a confusing answer choice.

## 7. Your First Instinct

Many people struggle with multiple-choice tests because they overthink the questions. If you have studied sufficiently for the test, you should be prepared to trust your first instinct once you have carefully and completely read the question and all of the answer choices. There is a great deal of research suggesting that the mind can come to the correct conclusion very quickly once it has obtained all of the relevant information. At times, it may seem to you as if your intuition is working faster even than your reasoning mind. This may in fact be true. The knowledge you obtain while studying may be retrieved from your subconscious before you have a chance to work out the associations that support it. Verify your instinct by working out the reasons that it should be trusted.

## 8. Key Words

Many test takers struggle with multiple-choice questions because they have poor reading comprehension skills. Quickly reading and understanding a multiple-choice question requires a mixture of skill and experience. To help with this, try jotting down a few key words and phrases on a piece of scrap paper. Doing this concentrates the process of reading and forces the mind to weigh the relative importance of the question's parts. In selecting words and phrases to write down, the test taker thinks about the question more deeply and carefully. This is especially true for multiple-choice questions that are preceded by a long prompt.

## 9. Subtle Negatives

One of the oldest tricks in the multiple-choice test writer's book is to subtly reverse the meaning of a question with a word like *not* or *except*. If you are not paying attention to each word in the question, you can easily be led astray by this trick. For instance, a common question format is, "Which of the following is...?" Obviously, if the question instead is, "Which of the following is not...?," then the answer will be quite different. Even worse, the test makers are aware of the potential for this mistake and will include one answer choice that would be correct if the question were not negated or reversed. A test taker who misses the reversal will find what he or she believes to be a correct answer and will be so confident that he or she will fail to reread the question and discover the original error. The only way to avoid this is to practice a wide variety of multiple-choice questions and to pay close attention to each and every word.

## 10. Reading Every Answer Choice

It may seem obvious, but you should always read every one of the answer choices! Too many test takers fall into the habit of scanning the question and assuming that they understand the question because they recognize a few key words. From there, they pick the first answer choice that answers the question they believe they have read. Test takers who read all of the answer choices might discover that one of the latter answer choices is actually *more* correct. Moreover, reading all of the answer choices can remind you of facts related to the question that can help you arrive at the correct answer. Sometimes, a misstatement or incorrect detail in one of the latter answer choices will trigger your memory of the subject and will enable you to find the right answer. Failing to read all of the answer choices is like not reading all of the items on a restaurant menu: you might miss out on the perfect choice.

## 11. Spot the Hedges

One of the keys to success on multiple-choice tests is paying close attention to every word. This is never truer than with words like almost, most, some, and sometimes. These words are called "hedges" because they indicate that a statement is not totally true or not true in every place and time. An absolute statement will contain no hedges, but in many subjects, the answers are not always straightforward or absolute. There are always exceptions to the rules in these subjects. For this reason, you should favor those multiple-choice questions that contain hedging language. The presence of qualifying words indicates that the author is taking special care with their words, which is certainly important when composing the right answer. After all, there are many ways to be wrong, but there is only one way to be right! For this reason, it is wise to avoid answers that are absolute when taking a multiple-choice test. An absolute answer is one that says things are either all one way or all another. They often include words like *every*, *always*, *best*, and *never*. If you are taking a multiple-choice test in a subject that doesn't lend itself to absolute answers, be on your guard if you see any of these words.

## 12. Long Answers

In many subject areas, the answers are not simple. As already mentioned, the right answer often requires hedges. Another common feature of the answers to a complex or subjective question are qualifying clauses, which are groups of words that subtly modify the meaning of the sentence. If the question or answer choice describes a rule to which there are exceptions or the subject matter is complicated, ambiguous, or confusing, the correct answer will require many words in order to be expressed clearly and accurately. In essence, you should not be deterred by answer choices that seem

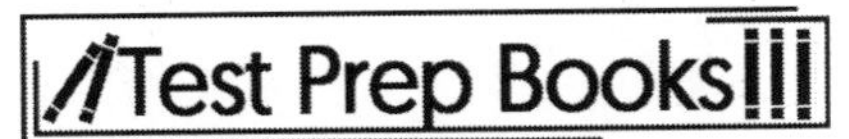

excessively long. Oftentimes, the author of the text will not be able to write the correct answer without offering some qualifications and modifications. Your job is to read the answer choices thoroughly and completely and to select the one that most accurately and precisely answers the question.

## 13. Restating to Understand

Sometimes, a question on a multiple-choice test is difficult not because of what it asks but because of how it is written. If this is the case, restate the question or answer choice in different words. This process serves a couple of important purposes. First, it forces you to concentrate on the core of the question. In order to rephrase the question accurately, you have to understand it well. Rephrasing the question will concentrate your mind on the key words and ideas. Second, it will present the information to your mind in a fresh way. This process may trigger your memory and render some useful scrap of information picked up while studying.

## 14. True Statements

Sometimes an answer choice will be true in itself, but it does not answer the question. This is one of the main reasons why it is essential to read the question carefully and completely before proceeding to the answer choices. Too often, test takers skip ahead to the answer choices and look for true statements. Having found one of these, they are content to select it without reference to the question above. Obviously, this provides an easy way for test makers to play tricks. The savvy test taker will always read the entire question before turning to the answer choices. Then, having settled on a correct answer choice, he or she will refer to the original question and ensure that the selected answer is relevant. The mistake of choosing a correct-but-irrelevant answer choice is especially common on questions related to specific pieces of objective knowledge. A prepared test taker will have a wealth of factual knowledge at their disposal, and should not be careless in its application.

## 15. No Patterns

One of the more dangerous ideas that circulates about multiple-choice tests is that the correct answers tend to fall into patterns. These erroneous ideas range from a belief that B and C are the most common right answers, to the idea that an unprepared test-taker should answer "A-B-A-C-A-D-A-B-A." It cannot be emphasized enough that pattern-seeking of this type is exactly the WRONG way to approach a multiple-choice test. To begin with, it is highly unlikely that the test maker will plot the correct answers according to some predetermined pattern. The questions are scrambled and delivered in a random order. Furthermore, even if the test maker was following a pattern in the assignation of correct answers, there is no reason why the test taker would know which pattern he or she was using. Any attempt to discern a pattern in the answer choices is a waste of time and a distraction from the real work of taking the test. A test taker would be much better served by extra preparation before the test than by reliance on a pattern in the answers.

# FREE Videos/DVD OFFER

Doing well on your exam requires both knowing the test content and understanding how to use that knowledge to do well on the test. We offer completely FREE test taking tip videos. **These videos cover world-class tips that you can use to succeed on your test.**

To get your **FREE videos**, you can use the QR code below or email freevideos@studyguideteam.com with "Free Videos" in the subject line and the following information in the body of the email:

a. The title of your product

b. Your product rating on a scale of 1-5, with 5 being the highest

c. Your feedback about the product

If you have any questions or concerns, please don't hesitate to contact us at info@studyguideteam.com.

Thanks again!

# Introduction to the CPHQ Exam

## Function of the Exam

The Certified Professional in Healthcare Quality® (CPHQ) exam is required for all candidates seeking Certified Professional in Healthcare Quality® certification. Earning this certification demonstrates one's competency in healthcare quality, dedication to the profession, and ability to improve outcomes across the care continuum. It also can add to a professional's credibility and can distinguish the professional in the field. The National Association for Healthcare Quality (NAHQ) designed the CPHQ to promote professionalism and excellence in the field of healthcare quality. To date, over 11,000 professionals in healthcare quality have achieved certification.

The tasks and objectives defined on the CPHQ content outline are designed based on a job analysis conducted every three years. This job analysis examines the practice and skills of professionals in healthcare quality. Professionals in healthcare quality are defined as those who have on-the-job experience in conducting and/or managing healthcare quality activities such as performance and process improvement, coordination of care, risk management, patient safety, population health, the analysis and measurement of data, performance and quality improvement, and compliance with healthcare regulations. Healthcare quality professionals use administrative, information management, and evaluation skills while performing one or multiple of these functions.

After the job analysis was conducted, those tasks deemed significant to healthcare practice along the care continuum, including acute care, long-term care, home health care, managed care, behavioral health, managed care, and other common care settings, were included in the CPHQ exam. It is recommended that candidates have at least two years of direct experience as a healthcare quality professional. However, there are no formal eligibility requirements to sit for the exam.

## Test Administration

Candidates can register online or via a paper application for the exam. The exam is offered in a computer-based format at more than 300 PSI/AMP testing locations around the United States. Some international sites are available as well. Test takers can take the exam Monday through Friday. Evening and weekend availability may be offered. A current photo ID is required to gain entrance into the exam center.

Candidates who successfully pass the exam will receive a certificate, identification care, pin, and information about recertification 6-8 weeks after the date of administration. The Certified Professional in Healthcare Quality® credential remains valid from the date the certificate is received in the mail through a period of two years beginning the on January 1 of the calendar year beginning after the exam was passed.

Retakes are permitted for candidates who fail to pass the test, although a new application must be submitted, and test takers must wait 90 days to reapply. No more than three attempts may occur in 365 days, and if a candidate fails after the third attempt, he or she must wait a full year to retest. Candidates with documented disabilities can receive accommodations according to the Americans with Disabilities Act. PSI must be notified of the requested accommodations at the time of application and scheduling at least 45 days prior to the desired appointment date.

## Test Format

The CPHQ contains 140 multiple-choice questions, of which, 125 are scored. The remaining 15, which are randomly scattered throughout the exam, are used to gauge their worth for inclusion in future versions. Of the scored questions, approximately 26% are recall questions, which require the test taker to demonstrate their knowledge of specific concepts or facts applicable to the field. The majority of the questions, 57%, are application questions, which evaluate the test taker's ability to interpret and apply given information to a posed situation. Lastly, 17% of questions are analysis questions, which require the test taker to problem solve, integrate information, or use their judgement regarding one or multiple situations. Test takers are given three hours to complete the exam. The following table provides the domains on the exam and the number of scored questions for each major domain:

| Domain | Number of Questions |
|---|---|
| Organization Leadership | 35 |
| Structure and Organization | |
| Regulatory, Accreditation, and External Recognition | |
| Education, Training, and Communication | |
| Health Data Analytics | 30 |
| Design and Data Management | |
| Measurement and Analysis | |
| Performance and Process Improvement | 40 |
| Identifying Opportunities for Improvement | |
| Implementation and Evaluation | |
| Patient Safety | 20 |
| Assessment and Planning | |
| Implementation and Evaluation | |

## Scoring

An unofficial score report with the pass/fail status is available at the testing site upon completion of the exam. Even those candidates who "pass" must wait to use the CPHQ designation until after the certificate and official results are received via mail. Unofficial score reports also include the number of correct answers. Raw scores are scaled based on the difficulty of the question, which enables scores to be compared across different exams.

## Study Prep Plan for the CPHQ Exam

**1** **Schedule -** Use one of our study schedules below or come up with one of your own.

**2** **Relax -** Test anxiety can hurt even the best students. There are many ways to reduce stress. Find the one that works best for you.

**3** **Execute -** Once you have a good plan in place, be sure to stick to it.

**One Week Study Schedule**

|  |  |
|---|---|
| Day 1 | Organizational Leadership |
| Day 2 | Health Data Analytics |
| Day 3 | Performance and Process Improvement |
| Day 4 | Practice Test #1 |
| Day 5 | Practice Test #2 |
| Day 6 | Practice Test #3 |
| Day 7 | Take Your Exam! |

**Two Week Study Schedule**

|  |  |  |  |
|---|---|---|---|
| Day 1 | Organizational Leadership | Day 8 | Practice Test #1 |
| Day 2 | Regulatory, Accreditation, and... | Day 9 | Answer Explanations #1 |
| Day 3 | Education, Training, and Communication | Day 10 | Practice Test #2 |
| Day 4 | Health Data Analytics | Day 11 | Answer Explanations #2 |
| Day 5 | Measurement and Analysis | Day 12 | Practice Test #3 |
| Day 6 | Performance and Process Improvement | Day 13 | Answer Explanations #3 |
| Day 7 | Patient Safety | Day 14 | Take Your Exam! |

**One Month Study Schedule**

|  |  |  |  |  |  |
|---|---|---|---|---|---|
| Day 1 | Organizational Leadership | Day 11 | Health Data Analytics | Day 21 | Implementation and Evaluation |
| Day 2 | Engaging Stakeholders to Promote Quality... | Day 12 | The IHI Simple Data Collection Plan | Day 22 | Systems Thinking |
| Day 3 | Leading and Facilitating Change | Day 13 | Identifying or Selecting Measures | Day 23 | Practice Quiz |
| Day 4 | Regulatory, Accreditation, and External Recognition | Day 14 | Measurement and Analysis | Day 24 | Practice Test #1 |
| Day 5 | Accreditation, Certification, and Recognition Options | Day 15 | Practice Quiz | Day 25 | Answer Explanations #1 |
| Day 6 | Service Quality | Day 16 | Performance and Process Improvement | Day 26 | Practice Test #2 |
| Day 7 | Gaps in Patient Experience Outcomes | Day 17 | Performance Improvement Methods | Day 27 | Answer Explanations #2 |
| Day 8 | Education, Training, and Communication | Day 18 | Implementation and Evaluation | Day 28 | Practice Test #3 |
| Day 9 | Developing/Providing Survey Preparation... | Day 19 | Practice Quiz | Day 29 | Answer Explanations #3 |
| Day 10 | Practice Quiz | Day 20 | Patient Safety | Day 30 | Take Your Exam! |

**Build your own prep plan by visiting:**
**testprepbooks.com/prep**

# Organizational Leadership

## *Structure and Integration*

### Supporting Organizational Commitment to Quality

It is a well-known fact that when the leadership team functions effectively, performance improves. As the central organizing body of the organization, leadership has an obligation to deliver all of the functions of administration, including:

- Ensuring cohesion
- Defining vision and values
- Creating and executing strategy
- Ensuring alignment
- Engaging stakeholders
- Developing talent
- Managing performance
- Building accountability
- Ensuring succession
- Allocating resources
- Crafting the culture
- Delivering results

The leadership team is the organization's center. The business's performance is dependent upon how effective the leadership team is. The leadership team must give particular focus to defining key processes, implementing them with efficiency, studying the results, and then redesigning the processes in order to achieve the desired ends more effectively. Additionally, strategic communication must be consistent and deliver the message in a way that results in organization-wide understanding. Leadership must be actively involved in daily conversations and be engaged enough to unite people around a common cause. This reduces uncertainty and keeps people focused. It also leverages the power of leadership decisions in shaping beliefs and behaviors.

Leaders take discernment and strategic direction and transform them into goals and objectives. Systems for performance accountability can clarify what is expected of people. Only then can consequences or rewards be aligned with actual performance. Ideally, each process should be simple, efficient, and responsive to the situation and needs of a particular organization. Where applicable, processes may also need to be globally adaptable. Establishing and optimizing operational performance is a journey that never ends.

For the best leaders, the goal is **transformational leadership**. Transformational leaders use four key characteristics—charisma, inspiration, individualized consideration, and intellectual stimulation—to inspire confidence and to encourage employees to visualize a better future. Transformational leaders question the status quo and coach employees to develop to their full capability. Ultimately, transformational leaders and their followers form a symbiotic relationship that encourages motivation and honesty for everyone.

**Values-based leadership** is a perspective on people, philosophy, and processes. Values-based leaders grant authority to their subordinates and lead by example. They believe in the ideas of liberty, equality, and natural justice. Some characteristics of values-based leadership are respect for followers, integrity, clear thinking, vision, listening, inclusion, and trust. Values-based leadership often produces social change. The needs of the followers are more likely to be satisfied, which may ultimately change the beliefs and behavior of the followers. Values-based leadership provides strategic unity and allows independent initiative.

**Mechanistic organizations** are those that have highly complex structure. They are extremely formalized and centralized. Employees of mechanistic organizations are encouraged to perform routine tasks and rely heavily on programmed behaviors. Mechanistic organizations are generally slow to respond to the unfamiliar. They provide fewer opportunities for employees to exercise initiative and generally suppress the individual differences expressed by leaders and followers.

On the opposite end of the spectrum, **organic organizations** are flexible and adaptive with emphasis on lateral communication. Organic organizations utilize experts and knowledge rather than position and authority, and they offer fluid responsibilities rather than rigid job descriptions. Information is exchanged rather than handed down as instructions, and fewer constraints are imposed on the activity of members, encouraging the expression of individual behavior.

## Participating in Organization-Wide Strategic Planning Related to Quality

Each healthcare organization develops a strategic quality plan in order to guide the organization through the process of setting the right quality initiatives. Without a strategic plan, the organization will jump from one temporary fix to another. Each organization must create a team of quality professionals who can be trusted to ensure that quality products and services are delivered to all customers. If the organization has only one person with the responsibility and knowledge of quality, that person will need to create and educate a team of individuals who can take responsibility for the management of quality within their jobs.

The strategic quality planning process consists of two phases: research and strategy. The **research phase** includes everything necessary to collect and analyze data before the strategic quality planning starts. The **strategy phase** incorporates the steps needed to develop the actual plan. Every initiative must be tied to the key business processes and their performance indicators. Without this step, there would be no real impact on the balance sheet.

The first task of the strategic quality planning team is to examine the existing strategic plan. All team members must understand all of the corporate strategies. The quality strategies they develop must align with and support accomplishing corporate goals. During the research phase the team will evaluate all of the quality initiatives that the organization has used in the past, along with those they will use in the present. They will research and evaluate the significance of tools like Kaizen, reengineering, Six Sigma, and project management. They also need to calculate the cost of quality and compare it to their desire to aim for quality awards.

The team will then determine the answers to these questions:

- What initiatives have been used before?
- What was successful or unsuccessful?
- Why were some of initiatives successful and others not?

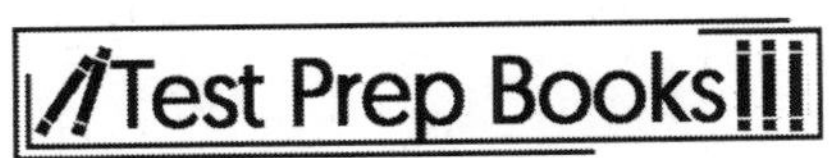

- What learning will come?
- Will the learning allow us to reduce the things that prevent success?
- Will it increase the factors that created success?

As a result of the thorough analysis, the team will eventually abandon some initiatives and choose others. They may want to revisit unsuccessful initiatives that they decide might have been done incorrectly or at the wrong time.

The initiatives must meet organizational needs, but they must also address customer needs. Customer satisfaction results can identify problems and opportunities. The performance of managers, executives, and employees can be assessed by reviewing customer satisfaction. The **voice of the customer (VOC)** can be obtained through customer surveys, interviews, and focus groups. The results of VOC can point out which quality strategies might help drive new product and service development. Service delivery and competitive positioning can also be improved by listening to VOC. Customer satisfaction levels cannot be determined until the customer's expectations and priorities have been stated.

It is also essential to involve employees when developing quality strategies. Employee input, such as voicing challenges, concerns, and ideas, can give additional insight to issues. It also ensures employee buy-in during the strategic implementation stage, which ties the quality development into action plans that impact employees directly.

**Benchmarking** is another way for the strategic quality planning team to decide how they can improve their internal quality processes, products, and structures. When they know what their competitors are doing, they can incorporate lessons learned into the development of their own quality strategies. During the strategy stage, the team must create their own vision of organizational quality and develop the strategies to achieve it. This may be a challenge since it is difficult to anticipate the future of healthcare. For this reason, some teams are more comfortable focusing on clear, short-term goals than on long-term visions that could be incorrect. The team must understand both present and future needs so they can align their organization with appropriate quality strategies.

Once the team has set their ideal vision, the team needs to develop and/or update their organizational quality policy. This policy must clarify the overall goal, mandate, and objective for quality. The quality policy should be a brief statement that shows the organizational commitment to quality. With this policy, the organization can ensure that all employees are aware of, aligned with, and support the organization's intentions regarding quality management. The team then creates an operational effectiveness plan, starting by developing objectives that will meet each quality strategy. Detailed action plans are then used to detail how the objectives will be carried out.

## Aligning Quality and Safety Activities with Strategic Goals

A well-researched quality plan will provide clear directions for the organization to move forward. Every healthcare organization begins with a goal of caring for the sick and encouraging the health of the well. Strategic planning moves the organization onto a specific track that will ensure that the goals are all accomplished. Although healthcare organizations improve the health of their patients as one piece of their mission, strategic planning enables them to develop a well-organized plan built on the stability of the team. It is essential that the organizational mission and vision align with the goals of nationally recognized standards of care.

The planning team must also ensure that quality and safety activities are in sync with the strategic quality planning process. Strategic and operational goals have to be reviewed by all team members. Aggregated data can then be scrutinized for trends that could become critical success factors. Identified trends are often used to create **key performance indicators (KPI)**, the measurable results that will decide if the goals and objectives the team sets can be obtained.

The **Centers for Medicare and Medicaid Services (CMS)** has taken the lead in the national goal of transforming health care delivery. That goal aims to "meet the person-centered goals of each individual in creating a health care system that fully engages persons and families in the design, delivery and evaluation of care." In 2022, CMS published the National Quality Strategy for Healthcare. The strategy outlined the objectives and outcomes for action to realize eight broad, interrelated goals:

- Goal 1: Embed Quality into the Care Journey
- Goal 2: Advance Health Equity
- Goal 3: Promote Safety
- Goal 4: Foster Engagement
- Goal 5: Strengthen Resiliency
- Goal 6: Embrace the Digital Age
- Goal 7: Incentivize Innovation and Technology Adoption to Drive Care Improvements
- Goal 8: Increasing Alignment

There are also six strategic pillars intended to guide the actions of CMS. Healthcare organizations and CMS must strive to ensure that each of these pillars is incorporated into the eight goals listed above. The pillars are:

- Advance Equity: remove the barriers to health equity that are inherent in our healthcare system
- Expand Access: extend the Affordable Care Act and ensure access to excellent and affordable healthcare for all
- Engage Partners: work with various partners and local communities to make sure that healthcare solutions meet their needs
- Drive Innovation: encourage innovation to overcome the problems within our healthcare system and make sure that healthcare is focused on meeting the needs of individuals
- Protect Programs: use resources wisely to ensure the longevity of the programs
- Foster Excellence: build inclusive, constructive workplaces and strive for excellence in every area

The National Quality Strategy was further enhanced in 2022 with the updated **CMS Meaningful Measures**, which identifies key target areas where measuring and improving outcomes will provide significant benefits for patients and their families while also reducing the burden on clinicians and providers. Meaningful Measures 2.0 has five complementary goals:

- Put patients at the center of making beneficial health care choices by focusing on patient-led quality measures and ensuring transparency.
- Utilize measures of quality care to encourage equity in healthcare and to close any identified gaps.
- Encourage improved quality measurement through the Meaningful Measures Initiative.
- Use additional payment programs and public reporting to support continued improvement.
- Introduce digital systems and advanced data analytics to increase the efficiency of quality measures.

The strategic quality planning team must establish and monitor methods to avoid or reduce the mitigating factors associated with all of the listed items, including high-risk procedures and patient-care services. When preventing mistakes, such as during surgery, both the goals and activities must be clearly defined in a strategy known as **mistake-proofing**. This involves developing the necessary countermeasures to solve any problems before they actually occur. Mistake proofing is designed to prevent issues that are identified in advance as to what could possibly go wrong. Steps can then be taken to ensure that they do not go wrong.

The data associated with implementation must be periodically reported to the governing board, in compliance with fiduciary duty-of-care regulations. The **fiduciary duty-of-care rule** involves assurances that the board members are acting in good faith, in a prudent and reasonable fashion, and making decisions that are in the best interests of the organization. This regulation allows the board time to prepare a prompt response or adjustment to any detected errors or concerns. Once any errors are addressed, the initiatives can be reintroduced, and follow-up comparison data are gathered. The organization's ability to adhere to this cyclical evaluation process is the best quality indicator for positive safety outcomes. The chart below shows a few examples of CMS objectives and possible outcomes.

| Objectives | Desired Outcomes |
|---|---|
| Improve support for a culture of safety | • Improved application of safety practices involve all team members, patients, and families and assure that individuals' voices are heard<br>• Organizations exhibit strong leadership that educates and empowers the workforce to recognize harm and increase reporting of errors and potential errors<br>• Consumers have increased access to understandable health information<br>• Expanded use of evidence-based services and primary care<br>• Disparities in care are eliminated |
| Reduce inappropriate and unnecessary care | • Healthcare organizations continually assess adverse events in accordance with evidence-based practices<br>• Healthcare cost reductions are attributable to the reduction of unnecessary, duplicative, and inappropriate care<br>• Disparities in care are eliminated |
| Prevent or minimize harm in all settings | • HACs, Provider Preventable Conditions (PPCs), and health care-associated infections (HAIs) are reduced<br>• Medication error rates are improved<br>• Falls are decreased<br>• Visibility of harm is improved in all settings<br>• Expanded use of evidence-based services and primary care<br>• Person and family access to understandable health information is increased<br>• Disparities in care are eliminated |

## Engaging Stakeholders to Promote Quality and Safety

Senior leaders recognize that engaging stakeholders at every level of program development increases their interest and commitment as well as the likelihood of developing a successful program. If this is done well, stakeholders will begin to invest in long-term support for the program. Hospitals generally have multiple methodologies for engaging stakeholders. Three of the most successful strategies are finding "champions," leaders who will actively and visibly support both the program's initial phases and its long-term sustainability; building strong relationships with stakeholders and ensuring that they are kept up-to-date and receive frequent communications; and clearly communicating the outcomes of the program under development.

**Champions** assist with program growth and development and encourage program stability. These leaders must be stakeholders with a significant commitment to the program who are also highly respected by their peers. Program developers will be able to rely on the expertise and experience of these champions for help with program planning and design. The champions are also extremely helpful in promoting the program and ensuring its continuation and sustainability. They also help manage other stakeholders' expectations. Program champions can offer feedback by identifying areas for clarification and by giving input on potential initiatives and will also be in an excellent position to help program staff understand how other stakeholders may view preliminary evaluation results. Champions can be drawn from many different groups, including State and national agencies, state government, the provider community, patient advocates, and patients themselves. Input from the provider community is particularly important during the planning and designing stages as they can give expert advice on the clinical side of the program. Clinicians can also become champions and serve as ambassadors to their patients.

Ongoing **communication** encourages stakeholder support. Frequent and direct correspondence between stakeholders and program staff ensures that stakeholders have correct and up-to-date information about the program. Because program staff are the key contacts for the program, stakeholders will have a direct pipeline through which they can discuss all questions or concerns. After a program is implemented, continued stakeholder support depends on regular communication about the program's successes, failures, and any new plans that are being considered or introduced.

**Managing expectations** to maintain continued stakeholder support is primarily achieved by communicating program successes and outcomes to the stakeholders. To be successful, outcomes must be reported from the beginning of the program's implementation and updated frequently. It is particularly important to consider what outcomes and measurements will be most useful for each stakeholder group.

CMS developed an emergency preparedness checklist for healthcare facilities that has 70 tasks and gives guidance for developing emergency plans. Healthcare facilities are required to have disaster preparedness manuals and protocols that specify the steps to follow in the event of one of the following:

- Weather emergencies (tornado, hurricane, thunderstorms, etc.)
- Earthquakes and situations with power loss
- Infectious disease outbreaks
- Bomb threats
- Active shooters
- Bioterrorism

Community-based organizations work closely with case managers, physicians, and other members of the healthcare team to coordinate care, so it is important to include these organizations in all disaster preparedness planning. Community organizations working at a local level can promote patient

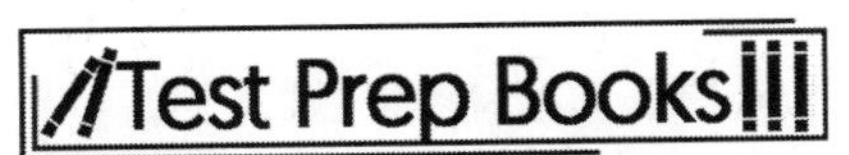

empowerment and self-management. These community vendors can provide a variety of services, including support groups or financial assistance.

## Providing Consultative Support to the Governing Body and Clinical Staff Regarding Their Roles and Responsibilities

It is essential that the leadership team of a healthcare organization work closely with the clinical staff regarding their roles and responsibilities. The three most crucial aspects are credentialing, privileging, and quality oversight. All clinical staff are required to meet stringent competency guidelines surrounding the specific competencies for each role. **Credentialing** includes allowing a licensed or certified medical professional to provide care within their scope of practice. **Privileging** includes an evaluation of the practitioner's actual performance and qualifications. In healthcare, for a particular provider to become eligible for reimbursement, they must meet a specific set of requirements regarding their educational preparation, clinical experience, and competence. The leadership team must maintain strict **oversight** of all medical staff by periodically verifying that each individual is qualified to perform their assigned duties. Privileging functions as an internal quality measure for patients. They can trust that the care they receive is from providers who have demonstrated excellence in clinical practice set by the medical governing board of the organization.

**Risk management** is the process of identifying actual (and potential) hazards and developing efficient, cost-effective plans to prevent them from occurring. A sentinel event is an adverse incident that has led to, or has the potential to lead to, a catastrophic outcome. Sentinel events require an immediate intervention. After any workplace accident or near miss, it is mandatory to complete an incident report. Within this report are the variables that caused or assisted the problem. Individuals involved are interviewed, the scene is examined, and management is notified.

During the root-cause analysis, the risk-management team utilizes the answers found in incident reports and interviews to determine the main cause of the sentinel event. The focus then changes from the problem to the solution and the leadership team collaborates with the risk-management team to dialogue about gaps in procedures, policies, workforce, and/or environment that need to be addressed. The primary objective in this step is to prevent future occurrences of a similar nature, while preserving the factors that did not contribute to the problem. The best changes to implement are feasible, efficient, and cost effective.

## Facilitating Development of the Quality Structure

In order to develop quality initiatives, the healthcare organization must designate quality-improvement councils and committees to build the foundation of excellence. The **American Health Care Association (AHCA)** was established in 2012 in an effort to improve the quality of patient care in post-acute and long-term-care facilities. This initiative focuses on the achievement of favorably measurable outcomes by March 2021 in four specific areas:

- 10% reduction in hospitalizations
- 10% increase in overall customer satisfaction
- 15% increase in functional mobility outcomes
- 10% reduction in the administration of antipsychotic medications

These specific changes will improve the quality of care delivered and positively impact patient experiences. SMART goals are used to tie the safety activities to the strategic planning process. Roundtable discussions with members at each level of the healthcare team often reveal gaps in care that need to be addressed. Conducting quality strategy meetings may lead significant insights that can be used in the quality plan. During brainstorming sessions, council members look for viable options to reduce variations in quality by eliminating unnecessary or wasteful process steps. As an example, a SMART intervention for each safety initiative may involve several options: hourly rounding on every patient by nursing staff; fall precautions based on age, history, and medications; and remote access to the electronic health record (EHR) so physicians may readily view status changes. Each committee can be tasked with creating realistic methods to integrate the plan into current processes.

## Assisting in Evaluating or Developing Data Management Systems

Providing exceptional medical care to patients requires that protected health information be safeguarded. The **Health Insurance Portability and Accountability Act (HIPAA)** of 1996 is a federal statute requiring all entities who care for patients to protect their medical records as protected health information. The portability portion focuses on protecting patient rights to maintain health insurance coverage in the event of a loss of, or change in, employment status. The accountability portion of the bill covers how patient health information is guarded. Medical records are to be stored so that access is limited, and strict confidentiality is maintained. HIPAA protections cover all documentation that could reveal diagnoses, treatments, payments, and any other related medical information. Violations of the HIPAA laws may result in severe financial and legal sanctions on the offending organization. Employees who violate HIPAA laws are generally terminated.

Advances in technology continually inform how personal health information (PHI) is entered, stored, and retrieved. Patients must provide their written consent before release of PHI. Healthcare organizations must make each patient aware of the protections and limitations to their PHI policies whenever possible.

With the advent of the EHR, data management professionals within healthcare realized that they must remain attentive to its advantages and disadvantages. The digitizing of EHRs has led to more efficient recordkeeping and increased compliance with documentation standards. It has allowed multiple user access. The leadership team must ensure the PHI is protected through multiple firewalls and gradations of PHI access. In addition, protocols and policies must be in place to prevent and detect security breaches. Accreditation entities also require specific strategies and policies to manage PHI. Any failures in this area are damaging to an audit and could slow or derail accreditation efforts. The leadership team must work continuously to ensure that the healthcare organization remains compliant by guarding all aspects of PHI.

## Evaluating and Integrating External Best Practices

Historically, **evidence-based practices (EBP)** are those that have been proven, over time, to yield the most clinically significant impact on healthcare quality and standards. Strict adherence to EBP promotes commitment and professionalism. Many different organizations contribute to the body of knowledge known as evidence-based practices. The leading agencies responsible for shaping the best-practice body of knowledge include: the Institute for Healthcare Improvement (IHI), the World Health Organization (WHO), the National Quality Forum (NQF), and the Agency for Health Care Research and Quality (AHRQ).

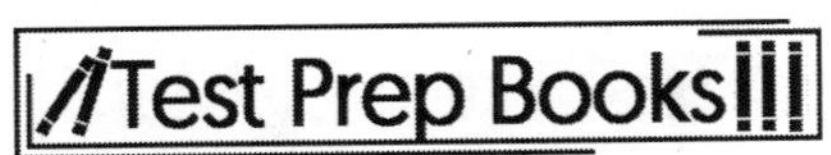

Combining their endorsed policies, procedures, and practices, these agencies have developed the structure for improving the quality of patient care around the world.

In 2001, the Institute of Medicine produced their "**Quality chasm**" report which detailed their major concerns about the differences in quality between current healthcare deficiencies and the ideal. The IHI later released a follow up to that report, denoting the six aims for improvement necessary to bridge the chasm: safety, effectiveness, patient-focused, timeliness, efficiency, and equitability. The goal of this report was to spark conversation around healthcare disparities and encourage momentum toward a culture of quality.

The NQF and AHRQ both endorse the utilization of quality performance measures to evaluate processes, patient experience, outcomes, and organizational structure. Both agencies also showed that repeated benchmarking (internal and external) fosters healthy competition that is needed to improve healthcare quality. The WHO implemented global efforts of quality and safety by initiating protocols on a larger scale. The WHO considers the importance of implementing healthcare interventions through a culturally sensitive approach. Since the inception of the Global Initiative for Emergency and Essential Surgical Care (GIEESC) in 2005, over 2,300 members and stakeholders from 140 countries have partnered together to improve access to quality healthcare around the world. This globalized healthcare organization has succeeded in changing the healthcare narrative to include underserved and economically-disadvantaged populations.

The **Healthcare Effectiveness Data and Information Set (HEDIS)** includes 92 measures grouped into 6 care domains and is used by over 90% of the healthcare plans in America. HEDIS is a powerful tool that is run by a private, non-profit organization called the **National Committee for Quality Assurance (NCQA)**. With HEDIS, it is possible to measure the effectiveness and quality of healthcare plans worldwide. Healthcare leaders understand the significance of using evidence-based practice to achieve better health outcomes. When the priority is placed on improving quality outcome measures, patients and all other stakeholders reap the benefits.

## Participating in Activities to Identify and Evaluate Innovative Solutions and Practices

**Innovation** is the process of developing new ideas, methods, or actions that improve upon a predecessor. Innovation in healthcare aims to improve current processes, polices, or standards that are outdated or inefficient in an effort to improve outcomes. Advances in technology have changed the ways healthcare teams research, retrieve, and spread information. It is necessary to identify current trends that will show where, why, and how to allocate resources. The leadership team must be able to use predictive analytics and move toward innovative solutions. Progress cannot exist without innovation.

One of the primary responsibilities of the leadership team is to remain informed of the fluctuations in industry standards. These changes can provide the foundation for continued innovation in each particular healthcare organization. To ensure that they remain up to date, some organizations may wish to create specific positions for leadership in strategy and innovation, while others may prefer to have the entire leadership team take on this responsibility.

Two of the most promising healthcare innovations of this decade include telemedicine and predictive technologies. **Telemedicine**, or **telehealth**, has reformed healthcare delivery across the country.

Providers can now conduct patient assessments, prescribe medications, and collaborate with other medical professionals remotely, via Skype, telephone, email, and secure chatrooms. Distance health eliminates the constraints of geography and mobility, and allows providers access to increasing numbers of previously underserved populations.

Predictive technologies, like patient analytics and medical informatics, help healthcare organizations remain ahead of the curve. Moving beyond the basic EHR, predictive analytics can create a multilingual medical record system. Although efficient, most systems do not communicate with each other. EHRs at two different offices may have software that cannot communicate with each other. This complicates the process and moves further away from a paperless system. Creating a standardized medical software or multilingual software that translates any data into useable information is required to create a more cohesive EHR system. Information technologists have started working on these issues. Other future innovations include the use of 3D printers to create prostheses, implantable devices, surgical tools, and instruments.

## Leading and Facilitating Change

Organizational leaders must have a specific skill set in order to lead and facilitate change. They need good business judgment, strategic insight, comfort with uncertainty, social intelligence, self-awareness, and people management skills in order to thrive. Change management must be a core competency because embracing change and taking risks are requirements for healthcare. The most effective method of facilitating change includes a combination of theories and stages of change.

There are many different theories related to behavioral change and the stages that an individual goes through in order to achieve lasting change. A few of these theories are detailed here.

The **Transtheoretical Model** focuses on the thinking process a person goes through even before the active process of change begins. This model has 6 stages:

- **Precontemplation** occurs when a person has not started thinking about change and may be oblivious to any need for change.
- **Contemplation** happens when a person is still not ready to make change but is beginning to think about it and may intend to make changes in the foreseeable future.
- During the **preparation** stage, the person is prepared to make changes in the immediate future and begins to actively get ready to make changes, such as through creating plans and setting goals.
- **Action** happens when a person makes clear and decisive changes.
- **Maintenance** occurs when the changes are sustained and become enduring habits that continue for a significant period of time.
- **Termination** occurs when the person has overcome both unwanted behaviors and the temptation to return to them.

Lewin's model of change has three distinct stages: unfreeze, change, and refreeze. Just as an ice cube can be melted, remolded, and refrozen, this model theorizes that the same process works with people seeking change. The first stage, **unfreeze**, involves looking at a situation and recognizing the need for

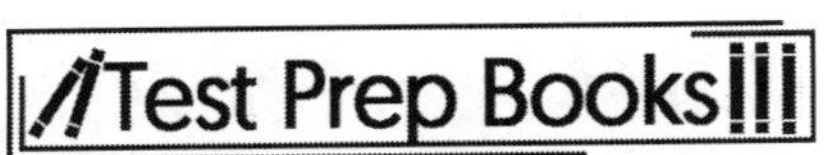

change. It is helping people challenge their current attitudes, habits, or behaviors, in order to make a persuasive case for why change is needed. During the next stage, **change**, new methods are sought, examined, and accepted. Finally, during the **refreeze** stage, these new habits and behaviors are solidified.

In Kotter's 8 step change theory, the first step is to **create urgency**, or to make use of a crisis situation in order to emphasize how urgently change is needed. The next step is to **form a coalition**, which is a team of professionals and family members who will work together to support the person making a change. After that it is important to **create a vision and strategy for change**, with goals and objectives, and then **communicate the vision** to all those who are involved in the process. The next step is to identify and **remove obstacles** that might stand in the way of a person achieving the goals they set. The sixth stage is to **create short-term wins** by recognizing and encouraging the small behavioral changes that are achieved. Once these small steps have been acknowledged, it is easy to **build on the change**, turning the small changes into bigger, long-lasting changes. The final step is to **anchor the change**, making the changes a permanent part of life.

As it applies to healthcare management, **diffusion** can be defined as the passive and unplanned spread of new practices. **Dissemination** occurs when new practices are actively spread; this usually involves specific and carefully planned targets and methodologies. **Implementation** occurs when those practices are adopted and integrated within a healthcare setting. The **spread** concept refers to the rate at which newly disseminated ideas or innovations are adopted and implemented. Leaders, acting as change agents, must always be prepared to employ these tactics to facilitate the changes necessary to improve the overall quality of care.

The **Diffusion of Innovation** theory states that innovations in healthcare spread over time, in five distinct and predictable phases: knowledge, persuasion, decision, implementation, and confirmation. Acting as the change agent, leaders must identify the innovators within the organization and appeal to them in the preliminary stages of the new project, providing knowledge about the concept. It is important to focus on the relative advantage, or benefits, of adopting the new idea over the old. Change agents must also consider ways to persuade innovators of the trialability of the concept, or it if can be implemented on a trial basis, without full commitment. It is essential to confirm that the chosen innovators will communicate their decision to implement the new strategy to stakeholders within the organization. As the use of the new concept or technology spreads within the organization, its implementation will phase out previous behaviors in favor of progress.

## Participating in Population Health Promotion and Continuum of Care Activities

Organizational leaders in healthcare must work diligently to develop activities which engage in healthcare promotion and the overall continuation of care of the populations they serve. An **episode of care (EOC)** is defined as all medical services for one individual patient, for a specific medical condition, from the onset of symptoms to the end of the final treatment. **Episode-based payments**, also referred to as **bundled payments** or **value-based care**, were introduced as a payment system in an effort to contain costs. This payment system is a contrast to the traditional **fee-for-service system**, which involves physicians receiving payment based on the number of patients that they care for, or the number of procedures they order.

A **standardized shift handoff** can provide a seamless transition between two different medical staff members who are providing care for the same patient. It can provide detailed and crucial information about the patient and the case. It also indicates official responsibility has moved from one provider to another. This provides a clear mechanism for accountability for oversight of specific tasks. All healthcare facilities have their own internal handoff protocol, with formal handoff training for new staff, ongoing training for established staff, verbal handoff protocols, written handoff forms, and consequences for employees who do not meet handoff standards.

**External handoffs** occur within two separate healthcare entities or during different transitions of care. Unless the two systems involved have similar procedures, external handoffs can be prone to errors. Standardizing a process may occur through a written checklist, a process flowchart, meaningful acronyms, or an audit tool for staff members to follow. Handoff errors can occur when established standard operating procedures are ignored, written poorly, or are too broad for the scope of the procedure. Errors in handoffs can also occur if medical staff are rushed, are unsure of the team members they are working with, or if they receive incorrect information at any time during the patient stay.

According to the CDC, a **transition of care** occurs when a patient moves between settings of care. A **setting of care** is any location where a patient receives medical care and may include hospitals, primary care and specialty care facilities, outpatient surgery centers, long-term care facilities, rehabilitation facilities, and even home health care. As the responsibility for patient care transitions from one healthcare professional to another, or from healthcare professionals to patients themselves, adverse events and miscommunications are more likely to occur. To avoid problems with transitions of care, it is necessary to have both clear and effective provider communication and complete patient understanding of discharge instructions. Patience and clarity on the part of healthcare providers is particularly important because patients are often confused and vulnerable during complex discharge processes.

Successful transitions require care coordination and logistical planning to reduce the risk of health complications that could lead to readmission, adverse events, an increase in healthcare costs, or a greater length of stay. A successful transition plan includes, at a minimum, scheduling and keeping appointments, effective medication management, and ongoing medication reconciliation.

## Communicating Resource Needs to Leadership to Improve Quality

When the leadership change agent identifies the need for specific resources, it is essential that the findings be communicated to the rest of the leadership team and the Board of Directors. Staffing and technology needs necessary to perform basic medical-related functions are all upper level decisions with a clear policy. Leaders must be effective resource managers in order to align the organizational mission, values, and goals with the needs of the employees and surrounding community. Internal staffing models can leverage the talent pool against the acuity of the workload of any given unit.

The AHRQ has developed a health information technology initiative to bridge the gap between technology and healthcare. Leadership must consider how social media and other technologies have become a part of the patient culture. Creating a social media presence increases the visibility of the health system and offers opportunities to publicize health information on a global scale. Once consent is obtained, health information in the form of emails and text messages can be sent directly to patients. Telemedicine, as discussed earlier, is also a rapidly growing option for patients with mobility issues or those in remote areas that have a difficult time attending in-person visits.

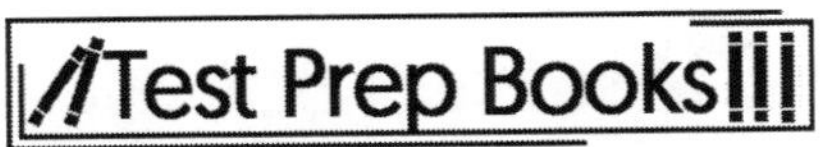

The **Health Information Technology for Economic and Clinical Health (HITECH) Act**, which was signed into law by President Obama in 2009 as a component of the American Recovery and Reinvest Act of 2009, supports and expedites the adoption of EHR-provided incentives to those providers who adopted the implementation and use of EHR systems through 2015. The HITECH Act increases the accessibility and exchange of protected health information and supports the electronic exchange of health information using EHR information. Under this act, patients or their appointed designees can gain access to their medical charts in an electronic format. This access enables patients to view their medical history and provides an enhanced method for information sharing among providers.

Providers and organizations must report security breaches related to electronic PHI as soon as it occurs, or they will face civil and/or criminal penalties. The HITECH Act also calls for physicians and hospitals that have meaningful use attestation to perform a HIPAA security risk assessment. To move between the three stages of meaningful use, providers must demonstrate the ability to function within each of the stages for two years before they can proceed to the next one.

## Recognizing Quality Initiatives Impacting Reimbursement

Historically, physicians have received payment based on the number of patients they provide care for. While the typical pay schedule generally consists of medical providers who are rarely paid incentives based on the care that they provide per qualifying health condition, recent changes to the fee-for-service model have been proposed. One of the most controversial forms of reimbursement includes the **pay for performance (P4P) method**. Although loosely based on quality indicators, the P4P model can also be seen as incentivizing physicians for efficiency, value, or reporting. It is a patient-centered quality-care model that encourages the development of a relationship between the physician and the patient. Patient perceptions of high-quality care then lead to continued collaboration with their provider. The core P4P model involves compensating providers for achieving specific quality standards or reducing healthcare costs. Quality measures typically include: patient engagement, health outcomes, care coordination, and patient satisfaction.

The current **physician value-based modifier system (PVM)** and the **value-based modifier program (VBM)** are quality-based initiatives designed to evaluate practitioners and provide payment based on adherence to specified quality indicators and cost-saving methods, rather than volume. While the P4P concept was proposed through the **Patient Protection and Affordable Care Act (PPACA)** of 2010, it was closely linked to **value-based purchasing (VBP)**. The VBP operates within hospitals, as a function of CMS, providing a financial incentive for reducing the DRG payments for Medicare patients. In recent years, the shift has been toward the VBM concept, with the stipulation that sanctions will be levied against providers who fail to meet standards of practice.

Proponents of quality initiatives suggest that P4P will encourage physicians to focus on quality over quantity regarding the provision of care. Those in support of this proposal believe that physicians will take more time with each patient, which will serve to improve all of the measures simultaneously. Opponents consider the initiatives to be punitive in nature. Arguments against P4P claim that policymakers do not take into account the increasing numbers of the elderly who will require ongoing care. Increasing patient loads without a compensatory rise in the number of attending physicians will result in poor outcomes across all quality measures. Others have reported concerns regarding the logistics of implementing the reporting technology. Overall, legislators, physicians, and healthcare leaders remain divided on P4P as the primary payer system in healthcare.

# Regulatory, Accreditation, and External Recognition

## Maintaining Awareness of Statutory and Regulatory Requirements

One of the major roles of the healthcare leadership team is to maintain awareness of all statutory and regulatory requirements and to ensure that the organization meets all of the goals. This role is detailed in the strategic quality plan, where key leaders may be listed as process owners or gatekeepers of individual requirements.

One way that the Centers for Medicare and Medicaid Services (CMS) helps consumers easily recognize whether or not an organization meets these goals is through its Overall Hospital Quality Star Ratings program, which it initiated in 2016 on its Hospital Compare website. In 2020, Hospital Compare and seven other health care comparison websites were rolled into a new Care Compare website and Overall Hospital Star Ratings became Overall Star Ratings. Each health organization receives an overall rating of one to five stars based on care and outcome measurements as well as a second rating of one to five stars based on patient experience. Care Compare also includes various other details about the health care provider such as services offered, office location, and various quality details and metrics. These ratings give consumers a clear and simple way to evaluate the quality of potential health care providers and compare them with other providers in their area. The ratings also impact the financial value of health care institutes and requires them to increase quality measurements if they want to remain competitive.

While strategic quality plans must be implemented from the top down, they will only be successful when there is an organization-wide commitment to meeting quality standards. It has become clear that the most successful health care organizations maintain high star ratings despite changes in quality measurements because they are committed to continuous quality improvement rather than simply checking off boxes in a strategic quality plan. Without a consistent feedback loop and a dedicated quality process, hospitals and other organizations will not have the data, analysis, or structure necessary to implement, maintain, or modify their strategic quality plans.

Hospital leaders should foster a high reliability culture that prioritizes safety, and several of its high-level corporate goals should be related to safety. When upper management has a commitment to safety transparency the programs are more likely to succeed. At hospitals where the frequency of patient handling injuries has been decreased, there are often administrators that encourage a culture of safety. Hospital administrators seeking to improve patient outcomes will need to consider how implementing safe patient handling policies, procedures, training, and equipment will all affect their bottom-line. Several case studies by the Occupational Safety and Health Administration (OSHA) have demonstrated that the initial capital investment in programs and equipment needed to safely handle patients can be regained within five years, especially when new equipment is paired with training and additional policies designed to maintain safety. Although there are significant equipment, training, and infrastructure costs are associated with implementing safe patient handling programs, hospitals that have succeeded have found that the economic costs are outweighed by the long-term benefits. Those benefits include:

- Reduced injuries
- Decreased loss of time and compensation claims
- Increased productivity
- Improved quality of work life and worker satisfaction

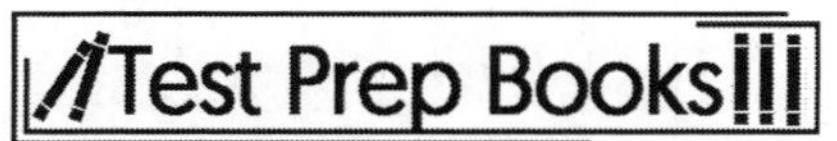

- Staff retention
- Better patient care and satisfaction

Management support should aim to include departments other than those involved in direct patient care, because departments such as laundry, maintenance, and engineering are also necessary to maintain patient health and safety. It's important that managers work with their employees and relevant unions prior to adding or improving on safe patient handling programs.

Because penalties for violating HIPAA are increasing, having policies and procedures in place to prevent privacy breaches is more important than ever. It is equally vital to ensure that these policies are documented and that appropriate steps are in place in the event a breach does occur. Leaders should appoint a privacy and security officer who is conversant in all HIPAA regulations and policies.

Healthcare organizations should regularly conduct HIPAA risk assessments to identify vulnerabilities. This will not only ensure that protected health information is secure, but will also allow healthcare organizations to address any issues discovered in the course of the assessments. Organizations should be particularly wary of email usage. Emailing information is allowed under HIPAA; however, encryption is highly recommended whenever possible. Wherever encryption is not feasible, patients must be advised of the risk of a breach when sending protected health information via email.

Storage of protected health information is another key area that must be addressed during HIPAA assessments, particularly when a healthcare organization uses portable electronic devices. For example, removal of such devices from the organization's premises should be strictly controlled. Each organization should make sure that any staff who use portable electronic devices are familiar with the guidelines HHS has laid out for their use, as well as receiving and documenting HIPAA training, attending refresher courses, and receiving training in any new policies as they are implemented.

A notice of privacy practices should be correctly published and distributed to all patients. It should also be displayed on the organization's website, and the organization should obtain acknowledgement of receipt from all their patients. The notice should be updated whenever policies are revised. Healthcare leaders should ensure that they are entering into valid business agreements with all business associates and subcontractors. Any existing business associate agreements must be updated to reflect the changes to HIPAA under the final rule, such as the expansion of liability of business associates. A protocol for investigating potential breaches of protected health information is essential. The **risk of harm standard** and the **risk assessment test** can be used to determine if a breach has occurred. If a HIPAA breach has occurred, it is essential that the healthcare organization document the results of the investigation and notify the appropriate authorities. Leaders must implement privacy and security policies, and they should sanction employees who violate them.

The **Affordable Care Act** was a turning point in U.S. public health policy. The Act introduced several revisions and extensions of U.S. healthcare law that were made to reinforce the previous legal framework and create basic legal protections that had not already been established. This included a near-universal guarantee of access to affordable coverage for lifetime health insurance. The fully-implemented Act reduced the number of uninsured Americans to less than half, providing coverage for nearly 94% of the national population. This reduced the number of uninsured individuals by 31 million and increased enrollment in Medicaid by 15 million people.

The Affordable Care had three main goals that it strove it accomplish. The first goal was to change the private insurance market by requiring companies to have competitive, reasonable prices, that would ultimately help individuals and small groups. The second goal was to expand Medicaid to cover US. citizens and legal residents whose family income was less than 133% of the federal poverty level. The final goal was to change how decisions were made concerning the medical industry.

To achieve these goals, the Affordable Care Act instituted the **Health Insurance Marketplace**, which uses **Exchanges** in each state to help families, individuals, and small businesses compare and enroll in medical insurance plans. The Exchanges dramatically simplify the process of selecting a health insurance plan by including side-by-side information on various types of plans, the cost and benefits of each, and the federal tax subsidies available to the consumer. Once a consumer selects a plan, enrollment through the Exchange is a simple process and there is frequent and clear communication regarding any additional documentation needed to complete enrollment (e.g., income verification for federal subsidies).

Additionally, the Affordable Care Act mandates that all qualified health insurance plans, even those sold outside the Exchanges, must meet certain federal standards. These standards include coverage of ten essential benefits: preventative and wellness services, outpatient services, hospitalization, emergency services, laboratory services, maternity and newborn care, mental health and substance use disorder services, prescription drug coverage, rehabilitation services and devices, and dental and vision coverage for children. Qualified plans must also meet other federally mandated quality and care standards. These provisions ensure that consumers will have at least a minimum level of coverage regardless of the plan they choose.

In addition to streamlining the purchase of insurance and setting basic standards for qualified plans, through changes to Medicare and Medicaid the Affordable Care Act gave the U.S. Department of Health and Human Services (HHS) and state Medicaid programs new authority to measure the effectiveness of new payment methods and new ways to deliver healthcare services to consumers. These changes are designed to increase the effectiveness and quality of healthcare services, make them more flexible to meet the diverse needs of consumers, lower the number of hospital admissions and readmissions due to chronic health conditions, and increase information transparency. If these programs work, it is hoped that they will become standards for the healthcare system as a whole.

The Affordable Care Act also instituted the **National Quality Strategy**, a set of goals, priorities, and levers that provide a roadmap of methodologies designed to improve healthcare quality and lower costs. It also created the **Patient Centered Outcomes Research Institute**, which is an independent, non-profit organization designed to provide information to patients about their health and the choices of healthcare available to them. One of its overarching goals is to make clinical research and, ultimately, healthcare more patient centered.

Another goal under the Affordable Care Act is establishing the Prevention and Public Health Trust Fund, a $15 billion initiative designed to support investments by communities that will improve public health. Such prevention initiatives include health centers in schools, activities to support oral healthcare, programs that encourage pregnant women enrolled in Medicaid to stop smoking, and adding Medicare personalized prevention planning. The Act has also focused on improving the quality of Indian healthcare programs.

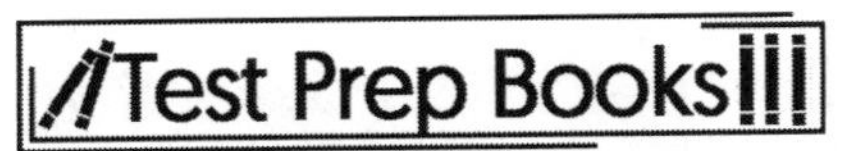

## Accreditation, Certification, and Recognition Options

Once a healthcare organization achieves the status of a certified provider through CMS and OSHA, the next step is to begin developing a plan to identify appropriate accreditation, certification, and recognition options. Potential employees and patients often diligently pursue healthcare organizations with specific certifications and accreditations, as they recognize the brand as a distinction of both quality and excellence. Competitors in the healthcare arena value distinction and recognition, since the standard of care is elevated and therefore signifies advances in clinical practice. Overall, the systematic appraisal of the care provided in hospitals, nursing facilities, and other healthcare organizations serves as a safeguard for patients and ensures that national industry standards are upheld. Continued certification or accreditation over time signifies an ongoing commitment to nationally recognized benchmarks for patient care. Although the CMS and OSHA inspections and subsequent endorsements are mandatory, not every certification, recognition, or accreditation standard is required.

It is important to recognize the difference between accreditation and certification. **Accreditation** is the process of evaluation of an organization by a third party according to a set of nationally recognized standards. One example is laboratory accreditation through The Joint Commission, which ensures that laboratory services are providing superior and accurate results. **Certification** is also voluntary and is typically granted to individuals, agencies, facilities, and programs. It is also conducted by a neutral third party and signifies that the recipient has exhibited the ability to provide specialized services. Obtaining the Certification as a Professional in Healthcare Quality shows an outstanding commitment to quality and patient safety.

For the leadership teams of healthcare organizations, one of the most important objectives is to develop a vision of the organization as a whole and to ensure that accreditation is maintained. Certification and accreditation entities have the unique ability to analyze processes and goals and can assist the organization in maintaining accreditation. The accreditation and regulatory bodies provide an unbiased, comprehensive assessment of the attributes of specific clinical programs and services of healthcare organizations. Additional benefits of accreditation and certification include risk management, increased access to funding sources that recognize a specific entity, accountability, process improvement, and business networking opportunities. As a result of the successful completion of the comprehensive assessment, any deficiencies are identified, and excellence is rewarded.

The entire process of achieving recognition is a time-consuming enterprise. Effective leaders have the foresight to consider which types of distinction are crucial in the infancy stage of the development of the organization. While considering the scope of the evaluation, the organization must be prepared to complete an initial self-evaluation. This critical step can identify gaps and redundancies in established processes prior to the site visit. An internal evaluation led by the leadership team can help in the coordination of survey teams, each assigned to streamline processes to meet the rigorous standards of the chosen entity. Policy and procedure manuals must demonstrate the typical lifecycle of a patient receiving care. Process flows depicting the application of current policies and procedures will also be necessary in an effort to confirm authenticity.

There are numerous options for healthcare organizations seeking distinction as excellent service providers. The most notable include the International Organization for Standardization (ISO), National Committee for Quality Assurance (NCQA), The Joint Commission (TJC), Accreditation Association of Ambulatory Healthcare (AAHC), Commission on Accreditation of Rehabilitation Facilities (CARF), Det

Norske Veritas & Germanischer Lloyd (DNVGL), Baldrige, and Magnet. Each entity has its own distinct application and survey preparation process, evaluation procedures and duration for its award.

The following table shows certifying agencies:

| Entity & Inception year | ISO 1947 | NCQA 1990 | TJC 1951 | AAHC 2010 | CARF 1966 | DNVGL 2008 | Baldrige 1987 | Magnet 1983 |
|---|---|---|---|---|---|---|---|---|
| Certification or Accreditation | Cert | Acc | Both | Acc | Acc | Acc includes ISO | Acc | Cert |
| On-Site Evaluation | Yes | No | Yes | No | Yes | Yes | No | Yes |
| Scope of Evaluation | Entire site | Site specific | Entire site | Site specific | Site specific | Entire site | Yes | Yes |
| Survey process | Yes | No | Yes | Yes | Yes | Yes | Yes | Annual |
| National Acceptance | Yes global | Yes | Yes | Yes | Yes | Yes global | Yes | Annual |
| Award Length | 3 yrs | 2 and 3 yrs by level | 3 yrs | 3 yrs | 1-3 | annual | annual | 4 yrs |

## Survey of Accreditation Readiness

Excellence in leadership requires a distinct level of expertise in vigilant surveillance. Once the leadership team has established which statutory and regulatory requirements are applicable to the organization, it is essential that the team members thoroughly understand the various standards of the accrediting bodies. Each organization will need to determine which entities provide the types of recognition that they seek and which will be the most valuable to their organization. Conversely, the leadership team must also consider the importance of accreditation in order to remain competitive in the healthcare marketplace. At each stage of growth, different forms of accreditation or certification become necessary. For example, it is mandatory for facilities that receive Medicare and Medicaid funds to obtain TJC accreditation to become eligible to care for those patients, but Magnet status is only established after several years of practice.

The leadership team must also take steps to prepare the facility and staff for the pending evaluation. Developing a culture of safety, customer-focused service, and clinical excellence is imperative. Discussing the purpose of the accreditation that the organization is seeking and how it will not only impact the company but also each department and individual employee, will bolster participation and commitment to succeed. Staff must also be made aware of the random nature of the on-site visit and the expectation that each individual employee be prepared to participate in any aspect of the investigation. It is ideal if the organization begins the preparation for the assessment within a reasonable time frame, in order to allow time to adjust to any changes in established processes and integrate them into the daily tasks of employees. Daily, weekly, and monthly reminders of accreditation standards and principles during staff meetings, in email correspondence, and on the organizational bulletins and screensavers encourages familiarity with site visit objectives. A simple motto to encourage employees to remember the rationale behind the site visit and to guide their preparation is essential.

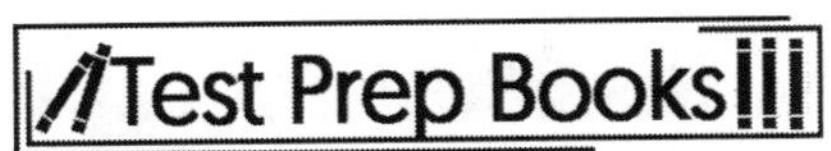

The next logical step in preparing for an accreditation site visit is to obtain a copy of the applicable standards, associated fees, and an in-depth self-assessment. Each entity typically utilizes an online application process along with supporting software and web-based evaluation tools to guide those preparing for the assessment. The leadership team oversees the accreditation process, so they must carefully research the standards in each domain and compare the requirements to the current policies and procedures of the organization. Organizations seeking accreditation from The Joint Commission must be prepared to review and demonstrate compliance with the National Patient Safety Goals. Top-performing individuals and departments can be recognized for their adherence to established guidelines listed in site-visit materials.

The methodical review of the accreditation standards and comparison to the existing organizational structure must be followed by a mock review. This step moves beyond self-assessment and presents the leadership and employees with intensive, periodic, and impromptu question-and-answer sessions. This type of preparation provides an advantage to the staff and reinforces their understanding of significant principles. Each simulated interview session can build upon its predecessor, increasing the overall score until the leadership team is satisfied with the results. If not required during the initial application process, the next step is to request a date for the actual site visit.

During the on-site assessment, leaders must remain impartial and have a working knowledge of the organizational structure, policies, procedures, and scope of the accreditation standards. After the opening conference, introduction to the leadership team, and discussion, the site surveyors will begin the actual interviews. In the case of a TJC evaluation, the assessors will conduct both individual and systemic tracer sessions. These roundtable discussions are a hallmark of The Joint Commission survey and include the use of an actual patient's journey through the organization from initial contact to exit.

Systemic tracer consultations are related to the review of the metrics associated with staff-to-patient ratios, medication administration, appropriate documentation, and National Patient Safety Goals. The assessment then enters the final phase, and the surveyors tour the facility and complete the exit interview with the leadership team. At that time, the surveyors will present their preliminary findings. Soon after the survey is completed, the final conclusions are disclosed to the management team of the organization. Organizations that do not receive any **requirements for improvement (RFI)** are notified of findings just prior to their public release. If any RFI are received, the facility will need to provide evidence that the citations have been addressed and corrected through the submission of an evidence of standards compliance report.

## Evaluating Compliance with Internal and External Requirements

As previously mentioned, the accreditation and certification process is multifaceted and requires significant preparation and buy-in from all members of the organization. The leadership team members must be equipped with the ability to monitor the organization's rate of compliance with evidence-based standards of practice. As the experts in clinical performance, it is imperative that the leadership team develops a method of gathering the data necessary to reflect adherence to the established requirements of the governing body. It is even more important for them to establish a method for data analysis and interpretation. It is through the clarification of the data that obsolete or ineffective procedures and policies can justifiably be transformed. For healthcare organizations in the position of providing clinical bedside care, there is a particular concern regarding medication use, infection rates, service quality, practitioner performance, gaps in expected outcomes for patients, and reportable events.

## Clinical Practice Guidelines and Pathways

When preparing for an on-site evaluation for accreditation, the medication administration policies and procedures of any healthcare organization are crucial. The leadership team, which includes physicians and the chief nursing officer, has the responsibility of deciding which clinical practice guidelines the organization will follow. When managing the care of patients, the safe administration of those medications is of paramount importance. Each clinician bears the responsibility of adhering to the five rights of medication administration, which ensures that each encounter involves: the right drug, the right dose, via the right route, at the right time, to the right patient.

With the advent of EHR, many healthcare facilities have charting at the bedside. This step is thought to encourage the clinician to confirm that all five objectives are met with the additional act of the bedside checks. The nurse is encouraged to review the medications as shown in the EHR, ensure that the EHR and medication taken from the medication cart or Pyxis match, and confirm that the EHR matches the medication retrieved from the med cart and is placed into the correct patient's medication basin. The data are gathered through the nurse actually scanning each medication and clicking the EHR in the appropriate section. In some cases, failure to perform this added task can prevent the administration of the medication and flag the patient chart for review.

Despite advances in technology helping to reduce medication errors, adverse drug events are still a significant cause of harm to patients. The ICU presents a higher risk of medication errors due to the nature of its more complex care. Additionally, such incidents in the ICU have been shown to more frequently cause serious harm or death to patients than elsewhere. Clinical practice guidelines are used to improve medication safety by highlighting strategies and changes that can be implemented in the ICU. Following guidelines and pathways results in fewer medication errors, improves quality of care and quality of life, and reduces risk and professional liability.

There are also several guidelines for infection prevention. The CDC guidelines for preventing the spread of infections in healthcare settings is the basic guideline adopted nationwide. There are two tiers of recommended precautions:

- Standard precautions should be used in all patient care settings. They are based on the assumption that each person may have an infectious disease, so a prudent person would use protection when dealing with body fluids. Standard precautions include hand hygiene; personal protective equipment (PPE); respiratory hygiene/cough etiquette; proper placement of patients; cleaning and disinfecting equipment, instruments/devices, and the healthcare environment; careful handling of laundry and textiles; safe injection practices; and healthcare worker safety, including correct handling and disposal of needles and other sharps.
- Transmission-based precautions are used in addition to standard precautions and address the method of exposure the patient may have.

    1. Contact precautions should be used with patients who have a known or suspected infection with an increased risk for transmission via contact.

    2. Droplet precautions should be used with patients who have a known or suspected infection that is transmitted via respiratory droplets (e.g., droplets formed when a patient is talking, coughing, or sneezing).

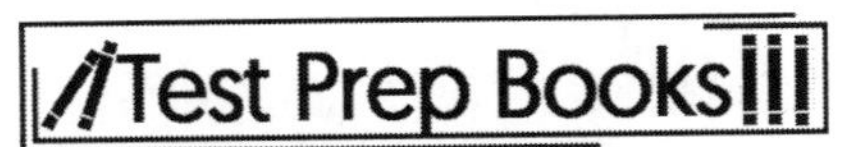

3. Airborne precautions should be used with patients who have a known or suspected infection that is transmitted via air from person to person (e.g., influenza, chickenpox, measles, anthrax, tuberculosis, smallpox, and SARS).

In addition to ensuring that all employees are educated about infection prevention, the leadership team must determine the best method of ensuring that the protocols are carried out. Leaders may oversee changes to infection control policies and processes and receive regular reports from infection prevention committees or teams. Administration generally also has input into who makes the determination of where patients are placed upon admission. It is not enough anymore to randomly assign beds based upon which floor has the most room. Careful attention must be made to avoid patient cross contamination.

Leadership is also responsible for ensuring that the following processes and policies are followed. These are key measures during site visits for all organizations and are often the cause of errors or sentinel events. In order to ensure patient safety each one must be regularly assessed, and policies must be reviewed and updated according to organizational policy. The healthcare organization must have policies and procedures that address the following:

- hand hygiene
- use of personal protective equipment
- respiratory hygiene/cough etiquette principles
- appropriate patient placement
- the proper cleaning and handling of patient equipment and instruments
- the proper handling of textiles and laundry
- safe injection practices
- safe sharps handling and disposal
- the steps needed to clean and disinfect the environment

## Service Quality

Leaders understand that service quality is one of the most important factors to monitor. It will always be necessary to make sure that all of the applicable quality indicators are met and that service to all patients remains at the highest level. Practitioner performance is directly related to the provider's ability to maintain a standard of excellence in clinical practice and service delivery. It is also imperative that organizational leaders work with departmental team leaders and managers to encourage their direct reports to consider options for credentialing. This is not only vital to the actual employee, but for the team, department, and organization as a whole. One of the best ways to accomplish this task is through ongoing peer reviews. Despite the fact that most managers are aware of the roles that each individual employee is supposed to play on their team, they may not be aware of how that employee interacts with other team members. It may be even more difficult for the manager to accurately assess the untapped strengths of the members of their team. Peer reviews provide colleagues with the opportunity to share constructive feedback about each other in confidence.

**Value-based payment** is a system originally implemented by CMS to increase accountability of healthcare providers and improve quality. Value-based payment assumes that quality is easily quantifiable, but measurement of healthcare quality is still improving. A challenge for value-based payment is that the high volume of data that needs to be recorded is time-consuming and might not always be relevant or helpful to patients. A study in 2014 reported that medical practices spend 15.1 hours per week tracking quality metrics for Medicare and other payers.

There have been efforts to implement EHRs to reduce difficulty of tracking data, but the solution isn't perfect. In many cases, using EHRs has simply changed the busy work from analog paperwork to digital data recording. One concern is that quality is largely measured by whether certain routine tasks have been accomplished. Those invested in the healthcare industry have pushed for a focus on patient health outcomes, since healthcare providers will assume greater financial responsibility under value-based repayment and other models. Additional metrics would then be necessary to reliably track such outcomes.

## Documentation

Because the healthcare industry is extremely high-risk, compliance is of utmost importance. Healthcare compliance consists of obeying various rules, laws, and regulations implemented at both state and federal levels that guide the healthcare industry and its practices. Compliance impacts every area of healthcare, but its most important functions are regulating patient safety, patient privacy, and billing. Lack of compliance can lead to fines, lawsuits, and may even end with loss of licenses if a violation is serious enough.

It is vitally important for those working in the healthcare industry to maintain knowledge of compliance practices; however, this can often be a complicated process as laws and regulations change. The following is a list of some of the organizations and federal regulations that set healthcare compliance standards:

- **Social Security Act (SSA)**: Lays out the requirements for Medicare, Medicaid, and various other programs for maternal and child healthcare (e.g., CHIP) as well as supporting the administration of some of the programs.
- **Health Insurance Portability and Accountability Act (HIPAA)**: Sets national standards for patient privacy and the protection of patients' medical records and personal health information.
- **Health Information Technology for Economic and Clinical Health Act (HITECH Act)**: Incentivizes the use of electronic health records and other healthcare information technology.
- **False Claims Act (FCA)**: Prohibits submitting fraudulent healthcare claims to the federal government.
- **Patient Protection and Affordable Care Act (ACA)**: Regulates private insurance, expanded Medicaid, and provides subsidies to make health insurance more affordable.
- **Drug Enforcement Administration (DEA)**: Enforces laws and regulations regarding controlled substances.
- **Food and Drug Administration (FDA)**: Regulates medications, vaccines, biological products, and medical devices as well as dietary supplements.
- **Office of the Inspector General (OIG)**: Investigates fraud, waste, and abuse for programs under the Department of Health and Human Services, particularly Medicaid and Medicare.

The **Office of Inspector General (OIG)** of the **Department of Health and Human Services (HHS)** fronts efforts promoting voluntary development and implementation of compliance programs in the

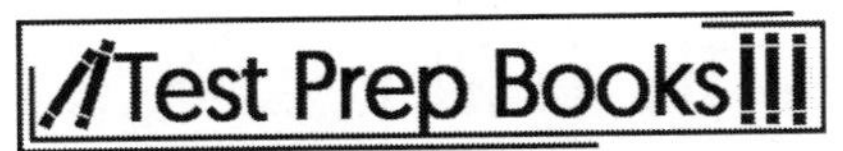

healthcare industry. Compliance guidelines for healthcare were issued by the OIG in 1998, which stated that comprehensive compliance programs should include at least the following seven elements:

1. The development and distribution of written standards of conduct, as well as written policies and procedures that promote the hospital's commitment to compliance, including adherence to compliance as an element in evaluating managers and employees;

2. The designation of a chief compliance officer and other appropriate bodies, charged with the responsibility of operating and monitoring the compliance program, and who report directly to the CEO and the governing body;

3. The development and implementation of regular, effective education and training programs for all affected employees;

4. The maintenance of a process, such as a hotline, to receive complaints, and the adoption of procedures to protect the anonymity of complainants and to protect whistleblowers from retaliation;

5. The development of a system to respond to allegations of improper/illegal activities and the enforcement of appropriate disciplinary action against employees who have violated internal compliance policies, applicable statutes, regulations or Federal health care program requirements;

6. The use of audits and/or other evaluation techniques to monitor compliance and assist in the reduction of identified problem area; and

7. The investigation and remediation of identified systemic problems and the development of policies addressing the non-employment or retention of sanctioned individuals.

The prevention of fraud, abuse, and waste in healthcare systems was improved by the development of voluntary compliance programs. Compliance programs are intended to develop a culture that prevents, detects, and resolves conduct that doesn't comply with healthcare law, healthcare program requirements, or the hospital's ethical and business practices. Ideally, a compliance program will show commitment to the compliance process and become a daily part of operations. It is important to use benchmarks that demonstrate the effectiveness and accomplishments from implementing the compliance program.

Executive leadership can, and must, lay out a framework for compliance that includes elements of transparency and ethical behavior. Ultimately, however, they can only set the tone. Compliance must be an organization-wide effort that each staff member upholds.

Most facilities use an electronic health record, which enables documentation to include time of observation, time task was performed, what was done, how it was done, and reaction to intervention. Documentation requirements are dictated by facility policy and regulatory guidelines. Two methods are used: charting by exception and comprehensive charting. Charting by exception means that besides recording of vital signs, only abnormal findings are documented. This charting method is somewhat controversial as so much information about the patient is usually left out. It is sometimes argued that this is the safer way to chart, as only what is deviant from normal is noted, and thus, there is less room for documentation errors. The normal is assumed, unless otherwise noted. This method also saves time, as less information needs to be documented, leaving more time for patient care.

Some facilities prefer a comprehensive method of documentation, charting everything about the patient, normal and abnormal, in a very thorough manner. This way, when the chart is reviewed, all details surrounding any event should be present in the medical record.

## Practitioner Performance Evaluation

Today, peer review is acknowledged as an ideal method to create a community that promotes professionalism and trust, while maintaining physicians' agency and upholding their duty of care. Peer reviews may be performed by various committees (e.g., ethics committees, credentials committees, and utilization committees), or by other reviewing bodies. The goal of peer review is to examine the conduct of healthcare professionals, and it is the primary method of performing such an evaluation.

The **American Medical Association (AMA) Code of Medical Ethics** states that physicians are obligated not only to uphold medical ethics and professional standards themselves, but to hold each other accountable as well. **Fairness** is a necessary element to any hearing that has bearing on the reputation or livelihood of a medical practitioner. Any individuals that take part in the peer review of others must strive diligently for a fair and objective review.

The Joint Commission outlines both the credentialing and privileging of medical practitioners.

> **Credentialing** is the process of obtaining, verifying, and assessing the qualifications of a practitioner to provide care or services in or for a health care organization. Credentials are documented evidence of licensure, education, training, experience, or other qualifications.

Credentialing is used to verify that data in an organization's documents is correct. An individual responsible for credentialing physicians uses multiple resources to verify this information, including a copy of the physician's National Provider Databank (NPDB) file, a credit report, and a criminal background check. The credentialing agency will also request a copy of the physician's credentials from the organization that presented them to verify accuracy. As part of an effort to lower rates of insurance fraud and abuse, the Affordable Care Act increased the credentialing requirements for Medicare and Medicaid, requiring the implementation of a repeat credentialing and confirmation process. The Joint Commission provides a detailed description of privileging.

> **Privileging** is the process whereby a specific scope and content of a patient care services are authorized for a healthcare practitioner by a health care organization, based on an evaluation of the individual's credentials and performance. A privilege is defined as an advantage, right, or benefit that is not available to everyone; the rights and advantages enjoyed by a relatively small group of people, usually as a result of education and experience. Privileges are specific to services provided at a specific location. Privileges can only be granted by the organization for services that are performed in the environment or organizations' location/building.

## Gaps in Patient Experience Outcomes

Patient satisfaction is becoming increasingly important as the cost of healthcare and health insurance increases and patients assume a larger financial responsibility in their personal healthcare. Additionally, it is clear that every provider and nurse handoff creates the potential for miscommunication and mistakes. As a result, patients wanting the best value from their healthcare services must now make

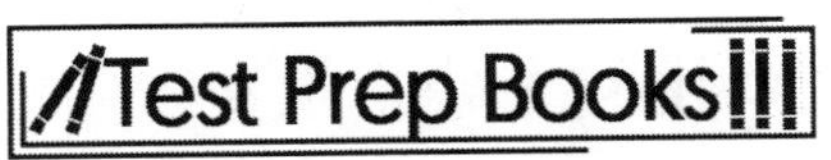

more involved decisions regarding their options and their care. It is critical that healthcare organizations utilize data gleaned from sources such as patient surveys, focus groups, team meetings, grievances, and complaints to meet these needs. Recognizing this change, the Centers for Medicare and Medicaid Services (CMS) have made patient satisfaction their top priority.

The **National Quality Forum (NQF)** is a non-profit organization devoted to improving patient outcomes by standardizing measurement and reporting. In May 2005, the NQF endorsed the **Hospital Consumer Assessment of Healthcare Providers and Systems (HCAHPS)** survey, representing the interests of healthcare providers, consumers, professional associations, government agencies, and other organizations. This is the nation's first reported, standardized survey to gauge patient views on their hospital care. The HCAHPS survey features 19 questions covering the following nine topics:

- Communication with doctors
- Communication with nurses
- Responsiveness of hospital staff
- Communication about pain
- Communication about medicines
- Discharge information
- Cleanliness of the hospital environment
- Quietness of the hospital environment
- Transition of care

As part of the survey, there are also three screener questions to guide patients to the relevant portion of the survey, five demographic questions, and two questions for Congressionally-mandated reports, giving the survey a total of 29 official questions. Hospitals may also choose to add their own questions to the survey, but these additional survey items are not reviewed or recorded by CMS.

The purpose of the HCAHPS is to make a standardized survey and data collection method available that provides a metric of patients' views on healthcare services. Before the HCAHPS survey was implemented, there were already hospital surveys, but there was no standardization or public reporting that would allow consumers to easily compare healthcare providers. Thus, the HCAHPS was necessary to provide a standard measurement of hospital care and quality.

The survey is designed to gather data from patients that allows for relevant, objective comparisons between hospitals. Because the survey results are available to the public, hospitals are incentivized to improve the quality of their services, while increasing public accountability through the transparency of hospital care.

## Reportable Events for Accreditation and Regulatory Bodies

An **adverse event** describes harm to a patient as a result of medical care or harm that occurs in a health care setting. A **never event** refers to a specific list of serious events or errors that should never be allowed to happen in a healthcare setting, according to the National Quality Forum. Never events include errors such as performing surgery on the wrong patient or leaving a tool or other object inside a patient after surgery. The Tax Relief and Health Care Act of 2006 mandated that the OIG report to Congress about such events.

Patient safety event reporting systems are one of the main methods of identifying adverse events and other quality of care problems. The general term for voluntary event reporting systems is incidence reporting. It relies primarily on the healthcare providers who were involved in a patient safety incident, a near miss, or who observed unsafe conditions to give detailed reports of the event. These are passive systems, unlike provider observation, chart reviews, or electronic notifications. Additionally, they are based on each individual's definition of an incident, near miss, or unsafe conditions, which makes them less reliable than active systems.

To increase the efficacy of incidence reporting, healthcare organizations must institute reporting systems with four main components. First, they must actively support staff who report incidents and vigorously protect their privacy. Second, they must make sure that they are receiving reports from individuals at every level of the organization, not just from a narrow selection of personnel. Third, reports of any incidents must be rapidly distributed to avoid a repeat of the event. Fourth, organizations must have a system in place for reviewing incident reports and finding solutions to the issues they identify. Recent developments that can assist with these goals include web-based systems, systems that are linked to electronic medical records, and specialized systems for specific settings (e.g., the Intensive Care Unit Safety Reporting System and systems that specifically report incidents involving anesthesia).

Simply having incident reporting systems is not enough, however. Concerns have been raised that healthcare event reporting systems focus too much on gathering reports and not enough on following up with action plans to prevent further events. Without a system for finding the cause of adverse events and creating solutions to avoid them, event reporting systems cannot adequately improve patient safety.

## Facilitating Communication with Accrediting and Regulatory Bodies

Communication with the accrediting and regulatory entities does not end with the initial evaluation. Maintaining an excellent standard of clinical practice is ongoing and never ending. At each level within the organization, there must be an expectation that the entire organization works toward individual and collective success. Once a specific recognition has been obtained, the organization must remain diligent in maintaining continued compliance. Leaders must be alert for changes in the standards and practices of the governing bodies and accrediting agencies they work with.

When attempting recertification, senior leaders must have current copies of all manuals that dictate the standards associated with specific accrediting bodies. It is also essential to review the previous assessment in order to ensure that all areas where the organization met or exceeded expectations will continue to do so. Areas of deficiency must be reviewed. In areas that were previously deficient, have enough improvements been made? Next, it will be necessary to observe changes in state and federal laws and amendments for necessary policy or procedural changes. Benchmarking must be done to determine if the organization compares well to competitors. This is important when reviewing the scorecard for the individual facility and for patient outcomes. The scorecard is a way for the public to monitor the status of any healthcare facility. If the competitors are equally accredited and have scored higher on quality indicators, leaders can utilize this information to gauge areas for improvement. It will then be necessary to prepare the organization to repeat the self-assessment, pretraining, and mock-interview process before the recertification process begins.

For the majority of organizations that provide direct patient care, The Joint Commission is the initial choice for accreditation. Once the accreditation is obtained, it is imperative that any failure to adhere to the agreed-upon standards is reported along with corrective measures. For example, any sentinel events involving the universal protocol, National Patient Safety Goals, or the speak-up initiative must be reported directly to The Joint Commission. It is important to note that although voluntary error reporting is a demonstration of best practice, it does not often yield actionable results.

When a sentinel or near-miss event arises within the organization, it must be reported as both an act of good faith and as a standard of evidence-based practice guidelines with The Joint Commission. Concerns can be filed anonymously online, faxed, or sent via US mail. It is vital that as much information as possible is provided so that The Joint Commission can conduct an investigation of the event. Once received, the incident will be cross-checked for other reported infractions within the organization in question. The investigation may begin with written notification to the agency or a site visit if the incident is deemed necessary. The personal information of the individual who files the concern can be shared without fear of reprisal, as the information will not be shared with the offending facility. Any resolution will be communicated to the reporting individual but, if there is no jurisdiction on the part of The Joint Commission, the issue may need to be referred to the state's department of health or legal authorities.

# *Education, Training, and Communication*

## Designing Performance, Process, and Quality Improvement Training

Despite a busy and fast-paced work environment, leaders at medical facilities must continuously train their employees. **Training** solidifies the existing skills of each employee and helps them improve in areas where they lack experience. Effective training programs identify specific areas where employees can improve in order to address them properly and allow every staff member to become both independent and competent in their roles. Effective training increases employee confidence in their abilities and knowledge, positively impacts performance across the board, and encourages the introduction of new ideas and methodologies.

Training must include information regarding personal and patient safety practices. The consistency of hospital policies improves when everyone is aware of current regulations for the organization and the healthcare industry as a whole. Studies have reported that one of the reasons nurses quit is due to poor education programs. Employees are more likely to remain satisfied if they receive training, because it encourages teamwork among staff members. Proper training helps everyone feel appreciated and that their hard work is being acknowledged.

Senior leaders must be able to create or replicate programs that work effectively with all learning types and are designed specifically for the organization. Training programs should be customized to address the specific needs of the organization as well as the needs of individual employees. This can best be achieved by including knowledgeable staff in the planning process for training programs. Their knowledge and experience are invaluable resources both for what should be included in a training program and for pitfalls to avoid. Leaders should also take advantage of technology by using new methods of teaching, such as simulation and just-in-time training. Screensavers and signs throughout the facility can also provide passive learning opportunities.

Leaders must be mindful that the efficacy of each program also needs to be improved. Inefficient or ineffective programs wastes money, time, and human resources. Leaders must assess the needs of the employee for a specific training and define the organization's training objectives before anything else is done. Surveys, patient feedback, performance reviews, and observations from team leaders or immediate supervisor can all be used to determine the educational needs of employees. Needs assessments for employee training should be performed to create the training program's goals, which will later help define performance expectations. Only after they know their objectives and what method will be utilized for training, can they move to the design, creation, and implementation of the program.

Methods of instruction can be lectures, written materials, SIM labs, just-in-time (JIT) training, seminars, or workshops. Some training will be short, and others will be extended. The location and times should fit easily into the employee workday. A training and development program is most effective when it is designed to meet the organization's goals and improves the skills and competencies of employees.

Finally, each healthcare organization must clearly outline the expected training outcomes. These can be measured through various methods, including performance tests and other evaluations. The results of these evaluations must then be considered carefully and any problems they identify must be corrected in the training program. Without this final step, it will be impossible to know whether or not the training has achieved its goals.

The leadership team of any healthcare organization is tasked with the development of strategies that improve the quality of current processes. It is necessary to eliminate waste, redundancies, and risks while working to expand currently successful strategies. Clinical excellence can only be obtained by developing processes that enhance the quality of healthcare delivery. Models of clinical excellence should be reviewed in order to determine the best model to utilize.

## Providing Education and Training on Performance, Process, and Quality Improvement

Healthcare organizations that seek to obtain and maintain accreditation recognize the advantages as well as the disadvantages of the experience. The majority of facilities are prepared to adopt stringent guidelines in favor of being added to the list of other esteemed organizations. The national brand recognition encourages competition in the healthcare marketplace and raises the standard of excellence for healthcare service delivery across the nation. State and federal laws are also built into most standards of accrediting entities.

The principles of both OSHA and CMS heavily influence the regulations developed by industry experts and provide the checks and balances necessary to sustain operational efficiency and processes. A positive review may also result in lower liability-insurance costs for the accredited organization. Since the application process includes a deep dive into procedures, policies, and risk management, unsafe practices may be uncovered that have the potential to prevent future patient harm. Once the final evaluation is published, facilities that meet or exceed industry standards are lauded for their successes.

Disadvantages are inherent in the process once violations become published. Although the offending facility is provided with a preliminary report, they cannot prevent citations from being publicized. Negative reviews impact patients' decisions to seek care at a specific organization in the future. One negative report, even if later corrected, can cause a facility to lose a once-stellar reputation and projected revenue. Employees and staff may face sanctions from a negative review as well. A failure to meet the expectations of current policies, procedures, or standard requirements could result in organizational restructuring or possible loss of employment.

Knowing these positives and negatives and understanding how employees might react to both, the leadership team must provide the education and training in a way that is non-threatening while fostering employee buy-in. There must be a component that explains what benefits the employee will

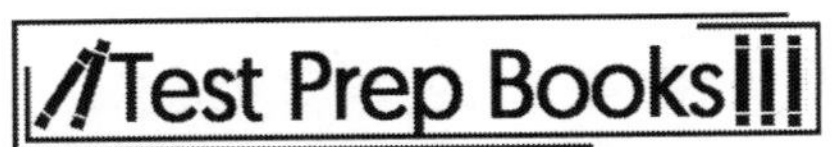

receive from participating in the training. Leaders must also incorporate change theory and project management processes into the training.

Training cannot simply be a leadership-oriented process, however. Unless it becomes habitual for employees at every level of a healthcare organization, training will fail to achieve its full effectiveness. Most organizational change is not maintained because it is not tied into the current culture, or it is so different from the culture that employees do not embrace it. These sorts of barriers should be identified early in the planning process and solutions should be incorporated from the very beginning of a training program. Continuous evaluation and feedback will help identify any continuing problems with implementation and any other issues that were not adequately addressed at the planning stage.

The **National Health Service Sustainability Model** is one example of a continuous quality improvement methodology that outlines four tools for identifying barriers to the continuation and success of quality improvement projects and improving the processes themselves. The first two tools are process control and performance boards, which communicate the results of improvement processes to both leadership and healthcare staff. The third tool is standard work, which is an outline of the current best practices for a given job. This outline also ensures that any improvements are implemented across the board and applied to all areas of patient care. The fourth tool is improvement huddles, short, frequent meetings that allow staff to anticipate and prevent problems, assess current performance, and build the habit of continuous improvement.

The leadership team developing each training must utilize all the tools available to deliver a quality education product. One particularly helpful tool that project managers can use to track their projects is regularly scheduled meetings where those involved in a project can exchange information about the project's progress. The project manager should often review several project elements during these status meetings:

- Task updates
- Schedule status update (behind or ahead of schedule?)
- Budget status update (under or over budget?)
- Quality/scope status update (maintaining desired scope/quality levels?)
- Current or anticipated issues (changes, risks, resource issues, etc.)
- Next steps

In order for the project manager to provide up-to-date information to the leadership team, status meetings should be held on a regular basis. The complexity of the project, the number of team members, and the amount of detail needed all affect the length and frequency of the meeting.

Successful meetings provide the project manager with timely updates on tasks and they let the team recognize milestone achievements, share information, and bring up any new problems. Unsuccessful meetings tend to fail in those similar areas. Typically, they are poorly planned, lack preparation, and don't correctly prioritize items. These meetings do not receive useful input from all team members, and often fail to manage their time wisely.

Dysfunctional meetings also significantly disrupt progress of the project itself. Aside from obvious negative effects to the schedule, budget, and quality, dysfunctional meetings also lower the project manager's credibility. Because the project manager is typically viewed as responsible for the effectiveness of status review meetings, when meetings don't go smoothly, or aren't relevant or efficient, the team members may view the project manager as incompetent.

## Performance/Quality Improvement Training

The effective evaluation of performance and process training begins with the determination of the most accurate and appropriate method of measuring success. The team may need to return to the data-collection phase if data are unclear. The analysis phase will reveal the data associated to the problems identified in the define stage of this methodology. If it is determined that there are several identified areas for improvement, the leadership team must scrutinize the data to verify the most crucial areas in need of improvement. These key areas will encourage the team to isolate the primary root causes for a deeper dive into analysis.

One of the primary tools utilized in the analysis phase is the **Pareto chart**. This quality-control tool helps to emphasize the most impactful problems in order to allocate the appropriate amount of resources to rectify the problem. The **Pareto diagram** is a graphic representation of the data collected to aid in the visualization of the frequency and root causes of deficits associated with the current processes.

Although the data may not actually meet the basic 100% with regard to total distribution, the data will clearly indicate the most significant variables. This display of the results will help to both quantify and qualify the variables. Pareto charts allow the leadership team to focus on operations that deliver on, rather than detract from, the value of the services provided. The data gleaned from the Pareto chart can be the foundation of the process-improvement initiative. Once the team is aware of which problems to address, the next step is to develop creative solutions. Through the internal benchmarking exercise, the team can look at departments in-house with similar issues and subsequent successes. Identifying the top performers in similar roles to participate in staff retraining is essential. Colleagues can normalize the new processes and demonstrate their effectiveness.

The competitive benchmarking option suggests looking to organizations with similar concerns that have succeeded in improving their outcomes. This is particularly effective among healthcare organizations that already possess or are seeking to obtain comparable accreditation. This task can be accomplished through reviewing the publicized summary of a competitor on the website of the governing body.

## Developing/Providing Survey Preparation Training

The leadership team will devote considerable time to the development and provision of the preparatory survey required for initial and ongoing accreditation. As previously mentioned, one of the most important tasks is to determine which accrediting bodies are vital and which are optional. The leadership team will begin by assembling the department leaders, top performers, risk-management staff, and medical governing board. The group must engage in roundtable discussions regarding their impressions of how each department has succeeded in their adherence to the organization's mission, values, and strategic goals. Wherever possible, established data from competing organizations is utilized and compared to current processes.

This strategy will help to answer the following questions: Where are we in reference to our articulated organizational mission, core values, and goals? Have current processes led to success or failure toward the realization of the articulated mission, core values, and goals? Which processes need to be changed, eliminated, or added to achieve our business goals? Where do we go from here strategically? How can

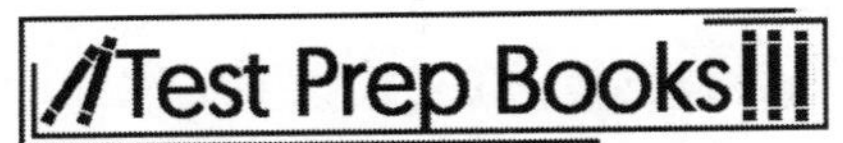

we get to where we want to go? How can we operationalize our business objectives as a healthcare organization? Do our proposed safety goals and activities align with established industry standards? The answers to these questions will guide the quality assurance team to prepare for the self-assessment required for accreditation.

Initially, the teams gather the basic timelines and presurvey guidelines from each accrediting body. For the majority of governing bodies, the suggested preparatory schedule allows for at least one year of current-process analysis, followed by status updates every three months. The correct standards and manuals must be obtained from each governing body and reviewed for new regulations as well as updates to prior standards. Previous surveys from the organization must also be scrutinized in order to ensure that any deficiencies or areas where policies or procedures failed to meet industry standards can be highlighted. Next, the committee will sift through the data to determine if any new areas within the organization need to obtain accreditation.

The team must initiate the actual self-assessment, with each individual staff member advised of performance expectations and measurement tools. This communicates individual and collective accountability for the survey results. This culture of expected excellence compels clinical staff to raise their performance to meet or exceed the projected outcome. The fundamental objective in these phases is to compare the organization's specified goals and activities to those proposed by the accrediting body.

Effective governance over survey preparation in the third interval prior to the on-site survey, or within approximately four months, involves documentation. Once the mock survey has been conducted, any gaps in services, polices, or processes will be uncovered. Process flows and policies must be updated and deemed legally appropriate. A separate but easily accessible electronic clearinghouse for the legally verified process and procedural documents must be created. There must also be evidence of strict policies regarding the method of approval regarding requests to update or revise documented processes and procedures.

Lead informatics managers must be named, along with their specific areas of expertise within the organization. Those identified leaders must be prepared to answer the questions of the review personnel and locate all documents associated with their respective departments. Actual staff must also be shadowed to prepare for their interactions with review personnel. Finally, within the month preceding the actual on-site survey, it is highly recommended that the organization conduct a second full-scale mock survey.

## Performance, Process, and Quality Improvement Information Within the Organization

The final task involved in the development of performance, process, and quality standards involves the dissemination of the on-site survey findings within the organization. This part of the process is the most critical facet of the maintenance of performance standards. There can be no uniformity in the application of the results of the new and improved processes if there is no dissemination of the results. If staff members are not made aware of the findings of the organizational self-assessment, they cannot be expected to adhere to them.

Once the survey has been completed and the organization has been privately notified of the results, the information is made available to the public. Similar organizations, patients, and even prospective clinical and ancillary staff can readily review the information. The Agency for Healthcare Research and Quality benchmarks for quality indicators remain central to the maintenance of a culture of commitment to quality and safety. This competitive benchmarking allows the organization to closely monitor and compare the progression of proposed changes to the current processes with their competitors subsequent to their separate on-site survey.

Recent changes noted in the 2018 TJC survey process indicate that the decision categories include: accredited, accredited with follow-up survey, preliminary denial of accreditation, and denial of accreditation. All results, favorable or not, must be provided to the organization in an effort to promote transparency, responsibility, and accountability. The leadership team must utilize all of the information contained in the summary to guide the discussions and generate the momentum necessary to maintain any changes to current processes. Follow-up surveys for those that have received a designation other than accredited will typically occur within two months. When preliminary denial requires the organization to provide additional detail, the organization must provide the information within ten working days. If approved, the organization will become accredited. If no progress has been made, the organization may request a formal appeal with the review board to dispute the findings.

It is necessary to include ongoing staff training after the successful completion of the survey process. Without this, continued quality improvement is not sustained. Leadership must do more than simply encourage clinical staff to personally initiate continuing education. In order to remain current on industry standards, employees must be directed to the website of the accrediting entity to complete specific continuing education credit modules.

**The Joint Commission** is an approved provider of continuing education credits by the majority of professional organizations, including but not limited to: The Accreditation Council for Continuing Medical Education (ACME), Accreditation Council for Pharmacy Education (ACPE), and American Nurses Credentialing Center (ANCC). Clinical leadership should also consider attending the webinars and trainings offered by the accrediting entity. The training modules review pertinent information regarding each standard, along with industry-specific rationales, and are essential for those involved in the survey process.

For organizations able to achieve accredited status through The Joint Commission, the journey is far from over. As previously mentioned, the procurement of accreditation for the entities that garner reimbursement are most valuable for sizable healthcare organizations. This is due to the federally deemed status that accredited organizations enjoy. For example, accomplishing accreditation through an entity with comparable or more stringent requirements, like The Joint Commission, enables a healthcare organization to waive the survey and certification process with CMS while continuing to remain eligible for federal reimbursement. The organization will receive a federal Condition of Participation certificate of compliance, either through governing entities like TJC or state auditors acting on the behalf of CMS. Despite the fact that each accrediting body has its own reaccreditation cycle, it is incumbent upon healthcare organizations to maintain a state of constant readiness.

Leadership must work diligently with clinical managers to encourage all employees to adopt a culture of safety. This can be accomplished internally through the dissemination of monthly risk reports to managers, to be shared during team meetings. Additional options include quarterly safety newsletters, rewards to top performers who exceed safety standards, and surveys regarding questions or concerns about quality.

## Practice Quiz

1. Which of the following terms refers to the "mood" of an organization?
   a. Environment
   b. Values
   c. Climate
   d. Culture

2. What is the difference between a mission statement and a vision statement?
   a. A mission statement focuses on day-to-day work, and a vision statement focuses on future goals.
   b. A mission statement focuses on future goals, and a mission statement focuses on day-to-day work.
   c. A mission statement focuses on day-to-day work, and a vision statement focuses on the process for this work.
   d. A mission statement focuses on future goals, and a vision statement focuses on the process for these goals.

3. Susan is preparing her team's department objectives that will be used to create individual goals and accomplishments for her employees' performance reviews. What should Susan ensure that each of these objectives includes?
   a. What the employee thinks should be changed in the department
   b. Specific, measurable, achievable, relevant, and time-bound aspects
   c. Professional growth, development, training, and learning opportunities
   d. Recognition and appreciation for previous performance and accomplishments

4. Which is the best data collection technique to use when there's a desire to reach a large number of people while trying to minimize cost?
   a. Focus group
   b. Interviews
   c. Observation
   d. Survey

5. What benefit can be gained by serving as a team leader?
   a. Communicating with other team leaders and directors.
   b. Being able to supervise and direct the work of others.
   c. Reaching the endpoint of professional learning and growth.
   d. Gaining knowledge about the business and operations.

**See answers on next page.**

# Answer Explanations

**1. C:** An organization's "mood" refers to the organizational climate, which can be directly affected by the environment, policies, behaviors, and process. Choice *A* is incorrect because environment is a general term that refers to the actual surroundings or conditions in which employees work. Choice *B* is incorrect because values refer to the ideas that guide an organization's actions. Choice *D* is incorrect because an organization's culture refers to the overall working environment, employer standards, interactions, and how work is accomplished.

**2. A:** A mission statement focuses on the day-to-day work that is being performed, and a vision statement focuses on the future goals and accomplishments. The mission statement supports the vision statement. Choices *B, C,* and *D* are all incorrect because the mission statement focuses on what is being done now, and the vision statement focuses on what will be done in the future.

**3. B:** Susan should ensure that each objective includes the SMART aspects: specific, measurable, achievable, relevant, and time-based. Without these aspects, an objective may not be met or the status could be unknown. By including the SMART aspects, there can be a clear understanding of performance expectations. Choice *A* is incorrect because all language should be well written, clear, concise, and specific, but without SMART aspects, there could still be misunderstandings as to what is to be accomplished. Choices *C* and *D* are inaccurate because professional development and recognition should be separate items contained within a performance review but separate from performance objectives. If a training opportunity is to be an objective for an employee, the item should be written as an objective, containing the SMART aspects.

**4. D:** A survey is the data collection technique that's best used when there's a desire to reach a large number of people while trying to minimize cost. Focus groups are interviews with small groups of individuals (typically three to twelve) and can be time-consuming to organize. Interviews are one-on-one meetings, are usually time-consuming, and require a skilled interviewer. Finally, observation involves visiting customers and watching them as they use or misuse products or services. Observations are also time-consuming and require a skilled observer.

**5. D:** Gaining knowledge about the business and operations, such as financial information, is a benefit of being able to serve as a team leader. This can be rewarding—both personally and professionally. Choices *A* and *B* are incorrect because communicating with others, supervising, and directing work are specific job duties a team leader would engage in and not examples of a benefit gained by serving in this role. Choice *C* is incorrect because an HR professional should never reach the endpoint of their professional development but should always strive to continue learning and growing.

# Health Data Analytics

## *Design and Data Management*

### Maintaining Confidentiality of Performance/Quality Improvement Records and Reports

**Data management** is the administrative process that acquires, validates, stores, protects, and processes data in order to maintain its accessibility, reliability, and timeliness according to the needs of the organization and consumer. Healthcare organizations analyze large data sets to guide their business decisions, discover the needs of the customer, and identify healthcare trends and opportunities to go beyond consumer expectations.

Companies develop data management solutions and platforms to handle the vast amount of data that healthcare organizations acquire. The goal with all data management solutions is to simplify the processing, validating, and handling of data, and overall become more efficient. Effective data management platforms enable healthcare organizations to manage large amounts of data from all sources to provide better communication with customers and retain customers longer. This is essential for healthcare organizations because they create and consume increasingly larger volumes of data. The best platforms provide companies a full view of their consumer base, which is necessary to gain valuable insight into consumer behavior and gain a business advantage.

In order to successfully make use of data management, organizations need to first have a goal in mind for the data they gather. A common problem for some organizations is that they may collect data well, but don't manage it properly to make it useful. Once they have a goal in mind, they can develop efficient systems to process, store, validate, and eventually analyze the data. Another problem that organizations run into is that their data might not be stored and organized in a way that can provide answers. They must focus each step of data management on their objective to make effective business decisions based on the data.

Healthcare organizations should strive to achieve the following data management best practices:

- Streamline the information flow for both traditional and emerging data
- Scrub data to ensure its accuracy and promote quality business processes
- Shape data to make it more easily understandable and usable

The **electronic health record (EHR)** is largely a collection of free-form narrative communicated by healthcare delivery. Insights, attributes of processes, prognoses, evaluations, and clinical observations are locked up in narrative. Unfortunately, narrative is not conducive to machine learning, data management, and next-generation analytics. It is only through controlled, structured, electronically-legible, and understood terminology that the value of clinical decision support, alerts, clinical rules, and analytics can be realized. Structured terminologies, also referred to as controlled medical vocabularies, provide the semantics of the concepts being conveyed in the electronic health record, and downstream in the data management foundation for analytics. Terminologies provide consistent meaning, promote shared understanding, facilitate communication, and enable comparison and integration of data. They are essential for interoperability among operational information systems, applications such as EHR sharing, and portability. Laboratory information systems also require these services as they process transactions in and out of the application. They need to translate from sending and receiving language sets.

One significant effort is underway to develop standard definitions for electronic quality measures (eMeasures). The National Quality Forum's Health Quality Measures Format recommends how health information technology (HIT) solutions should provide the data for quality measures in a standard format. The goal is to automate the measurement, feedback, and reporting of all current and future quality measures, accelerate the use of clinical decision support to improve performance on these measures, and align performance measures with the capabilities and limitations of HIT. Healthcare analytics are used to find inefficiencies in healthcare processes, identify items that can be improved, and improve implementation of resources. The lack of appropriate infrastructure, poor data integration, and privacy issues are all barriers toward adoption of analytics in healthcare.

Compliance with an organization-wide privacy policy is of paramount importance. Each individual with the potential to come into contact with protected health information must be advised of the privacy policy. The clinician must act as the gatekeeper, providing the information about any particular client's case to those specifically entitled to the information. In order to maintain the secured control of access to medical records, patients' information exists on a need-to-know basis. The **need-to-know rule** refers to individuals who must view the client's protected health information for the sole purpose of providing care. These individuals are to have access to the minimum amount of information necessary to perform the task at hand, nothing more. Only the minimum amount of information required to complete the tasks of caring for the patient should ever be released.

Signed, dated, and witnessed informed-consent forms that outline the types of information that can be released must be a mandatory facet of any treatment plan. Paper documents must be stored under lock and key with access only to the healthcare professional and necessary staff. Destruction of paper documents must occur through shredding, or by professionals proficient in document destruction. For electronic files and reports, the clinician must be diligent in the security of their desktop through the use of computer screen locks, shortened time-out locks, or black-out screens whenever the computer is left unattended. Computer access must also be limited. The clinician should consider placing the computer behind locked doors, with passwords that are changed frequently, multiple firewalls, and careful screening of incoming emails and documents to guard against computer viruses.

Whenever possible, electronic transfer of medical information, including emails and faxes, must be sent securely. The most effective process is to verbally confirm that the fax number is correct and stored in a secure location away from those without a need to know. Information to an individual should be limited to those who must have the information to perform their jobs. Any transmission of electronic medical records must contain a basic disclaimer advising the recipient on how to proceed if the documents were received in error, such as:

- This communication contains confidential information.
- If you have received this information in error, please notify the sender immediately by phone and return the original to the address listed on the form.
- Any distribution or reproduction of this transmission by anyone other than the intended party is strictly prohibited.

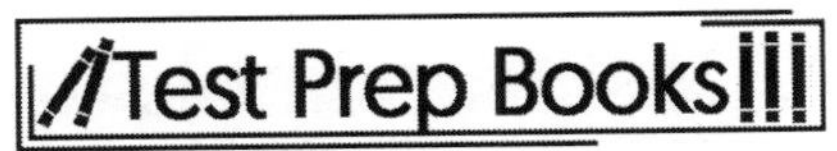

That verbiage, or something similar to it, should be added to all documents, emails, and other transmitted medical records. The clinician is the gatekeeper, ensuring that only the correct individuals receive the necessary information.

## Designing Data Collection Plans

The **Institute for Healthcare Improvement (IHI)** has a free data collection plan that healthcare organizations are encouraged to use. As stated previously, shamelessly stealing from the best practices of others is considered a best practice in healthcare. **Simple data collection planning** is one process outlined by IHI to make sure that the collected data is helpful, accurate, and can be gathered effectively. In particular, it strives to avoid collecting useless or unreliable data and also works to avoid processes that are overly costly or time-consuming. Simple data collection planning has the following benefits:

- The data contains current, accurate information that is useful for the improvement process under review.
- Common data collection errors can be avoided.
- The data collection process is streamlined to avoid wasting time and money collecting useless data or repeating unhelpful or failed tests.

## The IHI Simple Data Collection Plan

1. Begin your data collection planning by answering these key questions:

- What question do we need to answer—why are we collecting these data?
- What data analysis tools do we envision using to display the data after we have it?
- What type of data do we need in order to construct this tool and answer the question?
- Where in the process can we get this data?
- Who in the process can give us this data?
- How can we collect this data with minimum effort and chance of error?
- What additional data do we need to capture for future analysis, reference, and traceability?

2. Keep the following points in mind when planning for data collection:

- Seek usefulness, not perfection! Remember, data for improvement are different from data for research. Confusing the two can slow down improvement work. We need data that are "good enough" to permit us to take the next step in improving a process. These data are for learning, not judgment.
- Data recording must be easy. Try to build it in to the process under study. Use sampling as part of the plan to collect the data.
- Design the form with the collector's needs in mind.
- Minimize the possibility of errors.
- Provide clear, unambiguous directions.
- Use existing data whenever possible.

3. Develop your plan by answering the following questions:

- Who will collect the data?
- What data will be collected?
- When will the data be collected?
- Where will the data be collected?
- How will the data be collected?

4. When you developed a method to collect the data, test it with a few people who will be collecting the data and incorporate their ideas for improving the data collection plan.

- Be aware of the cost of collecting the data relative to the benefit gained from having it.
- Teach all of the data collectors how to collect the data correctly.
- Record what went wrong during the data collection so that learning can take place.
- Audit the data as it comes in for accuracy and completeness. Correct errors early.

## Measuring Development

Once the mission, goals, and values of a healthcare system have been evaluated, the leadership team creates a project charter. The project charter is specifically defined to serve as a written file that is a roadmap for process improvement. This written agreement usually includes the primary reason for the project, the goal and scope of the project, expected budget, and roles of each member of the team. Measurement is an essential part of testing and introducing changes. By using a variety of measures, a team can identify if the changes being made will be an improvement.

**Outcome measures** tell the organization how the system impacts the health and wellbeing of patients and shows the impacts on other stakeholders such as payers, employees, or the community. Some examples of outcome measures are:

- For diabetes: Average hemoglobin A1c level for diabetic patients
- For access: Number of days to the third next available appointment
- For critical care: Intensive Care Unit (ICU) percent unadjusted mortality
- For medication systems: Adverse drug events per 1,000 doses

**Process measures** indicate how well the parts of a system function and whether the team is making steady improvements. Examples of process measures include the following:

- For diabetes: Percentage of patients whose hemoglobin A1c level was measured twice in the last twelve months
- For access: Average daily clinician hours available for appointments
- For critical care: Percent of patients fully attended to during scheduled proactive rounding

**Balancing measures** examine a system from all sides to ensure that changes intended to fix one problem do not cause new problems elsewhere. A couple examples of balancing measures are:

- For reducing time patients spend on a ventilator after surgery: Make sure reintubation rates are not increasing
- For reducing patients' length of stay in the hospital: Make sure readmission rates are not increasing

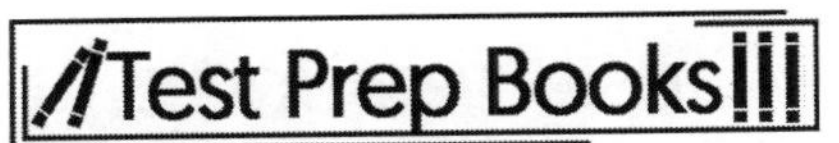

The leadership team must decide where to set the thresholds on their goals and objectives. Benchmarking with competitors and national organizations is a good starting point. Literature review for pertinent data will also give clues where the best thresholds need to be set. As an example, numerous studies have been done on C section rates, so when looking at these rates within an organization, a standard threshold limit can be easily determined. Similarly, infection rates, patient satisfaction, and readmission rates are easily located for benchmarking.

## Tools & Techniques

As stated earlier there are numerous internet sites where quality tools, plans, processes and guidelines are free to use. Using these tools helps to standardize the quality process and decreases the time spent collecting data. The leadership team is frequently tasked with gathering and compiling health-related data, validating, analyzing, and drawing specific conclusions regarding how to address noted deficiencies. The task at this stage is to select the most appropriate tools for gathering data as well as the tools used to analyze the data once collected.

Data can be either quantitative (numerical), or qualitative (descriptive). Quantitative data can be either continuous or discrete. **Discrete data** has finite values that can be counted. **Continuous data** has an infinite number of steps, forming a continuum with up to infinite precision. Some examples of discrete data include the number of children in a household, number of languages a person speaks, and number of people sleeping in statistics class; there may only be certain numbers of these (i.e. there cannot be one and a half people sleeping in class). Some examples of continuous data include the height of children, mass of cars, speed of trains. For example, a child's height could be 4.5 feet, or it might actually be 4.50003 feet.

There are seven fundamental tools used to evaluate quality, developed by a professor of engineering at Tokyo University named Kaoru Ishikawa.

The seven indispensable tools are:

1. **Cause-and-effect diagram** (also known as an Ishikawa or fishbone chart): A chart which identifies several possible causes for an issue and sorts them into useful categories.

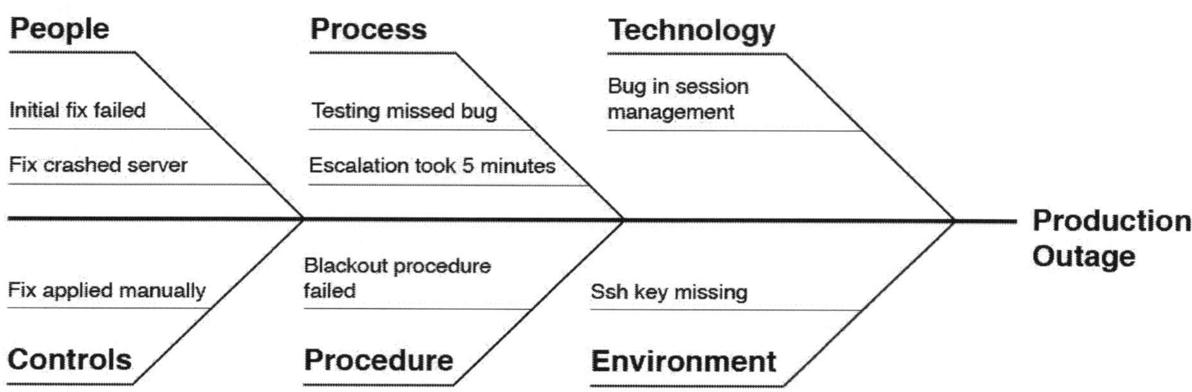


2. **Check sheet**: An organized form used to collect and analyze data; a general-purpose tool that can be used for a wide range of activities.

3. **Control chart**: A graph used to study how a process changes over time. A control chart begins with a time series graph. Control charts use a central line as a visual reference to aid in identifying shifts and trends. This is known as the process location. Upper and lower control limits (UCL and LCL), also referred to as the process dispersion, are made from available data and placed equal distances from the central line.

4. **Histogram**: The graph used most often to show frequency distributions, or how often each different value in a data set occurs.

5. **Pareto chart**: A bar graph that illustrates which factors have the most significant impact. Also called a distribution diagram.

## Example of a Pareto Chart

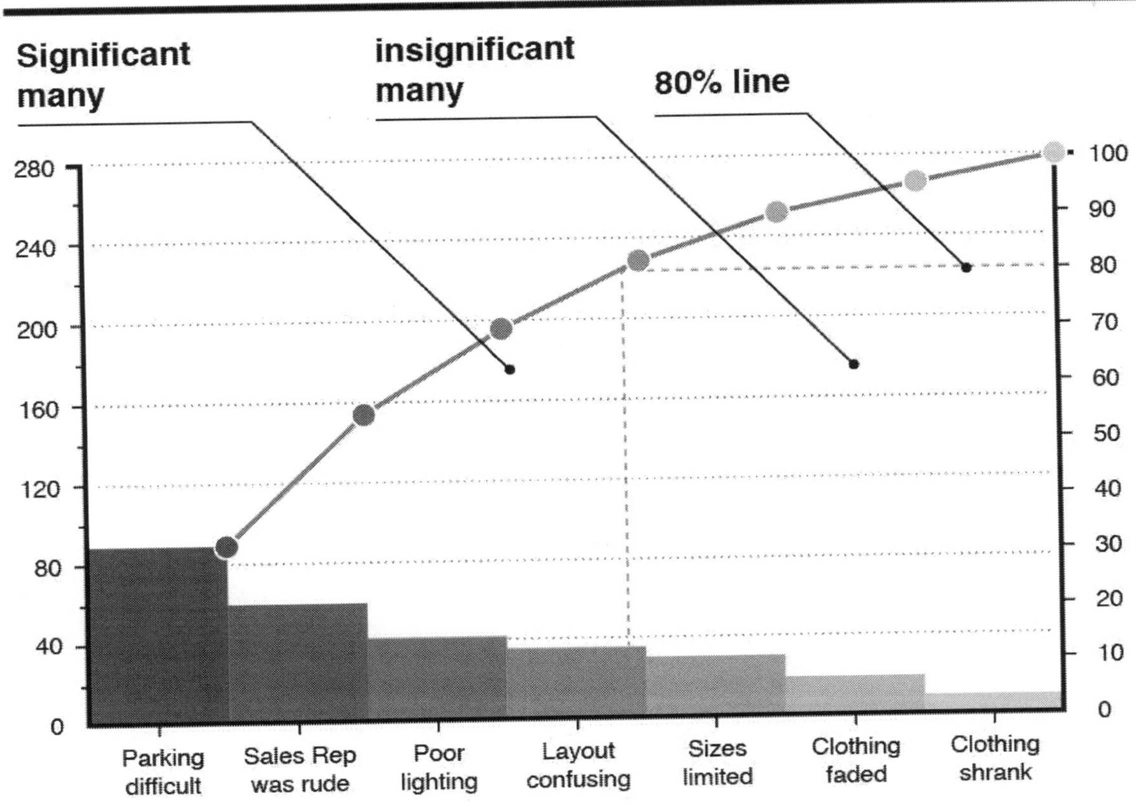


6. **Scatter diagram**: A graph that combines pairs of numerical data, using one variable per axis, to identify relationships in data sets.

7. **Stratification**: A technique that separates data gathered from a variety of sources so that patterns can be seen.

## Example of a Stratification

| Day | Mon | Tue | Wed | Thu | Fri | Sat | Sun |
|---|---|---|---|---|---|---|---|
| Frequency - Late in Office | *4* | *2* | *1* | *0* | *0* | *0* | *0* |

In addition to the basic 7, there are numerous other types of quality tools available for use. Free samples of the five why's, Gantt charts, x bar and R charts, z score, and others are all available on quality websites.

## Sampling Methodology

**Bias** occurs when the estimated result of your analysis is different from the true value of the statistic you are measuring. There are several reasons bias might be present, including sampling errors, measurement errors, or unrepresentative samples. **Sampling error** is the tendency of sample statistics to not perfectly represent the population. Error does not necessarily mean there was a human error or mistake. Even with a relatively large sample, some small amount of sampling error will still be present, because it's only part of the population. If a statistic is completely unbiased, the average of all statistics from all samples would average the true population parameter.

**Measurement error** occurs when the data gathered does not match the real values. For example, you might survey several people to find whether they support or oppose a bill. However, if the survey is worded poorly, some individuals may unintentionally respond with the opposite of their position. There are several sources of measurement error in statistics, including how a question is presented, the phrasing in a questionnaire, the method used for gathering data from respondents, and the surveyor's record-keeping system.

Sampling methods can be classified into two categories: probability and nonprobability.

## Probability Sampling

**Probability sampling** is when a small group, or sample, is randomly selected from a larger group or population. The key element of probability sampling is that every member of the large group has a known and equal chance of being selected for the sample group. This ensures that any information gathered about the sample group will provide accurate statistical inferences about the larger population.

## Simple Random Sampling (SRS)

**Simple random samples** are designed to provide an unbiased analysis of a larger population. To make sure that the random sample truly is random, it is vital that every member of the larger population is equally likely to be selected for the sample group.

## Stratified Sampling

**Stratified sampling** is used when a researcher wants to make sure that every group in a population is accurately represented in the sample group. To do this, the larger population is first divided into **strata**, or groups, based on a variety of variables, depending on the traits the researcher is examining. These traits can include age, gender, ethnicity, income bracket, job role, etc. Simple random sampling or systematic sampling is then used to draw the members of the sample group from each stratum. This methodology is especially helpful when analyzing a heterogenous population that can easily be divided into fairly uniform strata.

## Cluster Sampling

**Cluster sampling** divides populations into heterogenous groups called **clusters** that, ideally, have characteristics similar to those of the larger population. (Note that clusters are very different from strata – clusters should be heterogenous and represent the population as a whole while strata should be homogenous and represent only a portion of the population.) Random samples are obtained from a

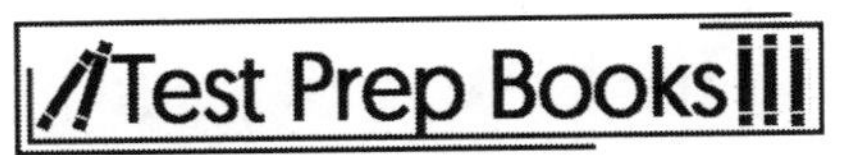

limited number of these clusters. While this method is useful for obtaining data from large or widespread populations, it does have two weaknesses. First, it is very difficult to determine whether or not a cluster accurately represents the entire population. Second, clusters may be dramatically different from each other, which could potentially skew the gathered data.

### Systematic Sampling

**Systematic sampling** is a probability sampling method which selects samples members from the population using a random start point and a recurring interval. This is called the sampling interval, which is calculated by dividing the population size by the desired sample size. For example, to sample 125 people out of 1,000, every eighth member of the population would be selected for the sample. For systematic sampling to be considered random, the start point must also be random and the interval must be decided before sampling. It is also important to make sure that there are no hidden or underlying patterns in the population list.

### Multistage Sampling

**Multi-stage sampling** also divides a population into clusters; however, unlike cluster sampling, the clusters in multi-stage sampling are further subdivided into smaller groups across multiple stages of sampling. This is also known as multi-stage cluster sampling. This sampling method takes large clusters of a population and divides them into smaller clusters in multiple steps to simplify the data collection process. If the same sample size is considered, multi-stage sampling is not as accurate as simple random sampling, but it reduces the cost and time requirements of data collection.

### Non-Probability Sampling

**Non-probability sampling** should be avoided because it introduces many potentially biased sources and it does not accurately represent the population as a whole. Instead of random samples, it uses voluntary samples and haphazard (convenience) samples. These kinds of samples are selected by hand, not at random, and thus they cannot be explained statistically. These common mistakes have disastrous results on the accuracy of sampling.

Projects targeting the improvement of defective processes in healthcare service delivery will require the collection of raw data at various points in the process. Once the project charter has been developed and the appropriate analytical tools have been chosen, the project management team will need to determine how often to collect the data in order to confirm that the appropriate amount of information has been gathered. This step entails asking several fundamental questions. Some of the most crucial include: Where will the data come from? How will we gather the data that we need? What are acceptable intervals within which to collect the necessary data? How will we know when we have what we need?

## Identifying or Selecting Measures

There are three types of quality measures that are used to evaluate and compare healthcare organizations: structural measures, process measures, and outcome measures. **Structural measures** indicate the healthcare organization's resources for providing quality care. In particular, it focuses on features such as the organization's capacity, systems, and processes. For example, a structural measure might compare the ratio of nurses to patients, the percentage of physicians who are board-certified, whether or not the organization maintains registers of patients with certain conditions, and what type of electronic medical record system the organization uses.

**Process measures** review the effectiveness of patient care and are the most common publicly reported healthcare quality measure. They focus on the healthcare activities actually done for patients and are often based on best practice recommendations for various procedures and conditions. For example, a process measure might track the percentage of women who get regular mammograms, the percentage of diabetes patients with controlled diabetes, or the percentage of patients with hypertension who get regular blood pressure checks. Process measures give patients an easy way to find out what treatment they will receive based on their condition, thus educating the patients and encouraging compliance with their treatment plans.

**Outcome measures** look at a healthcare organization's outcomes of care, which are the results of the patient's healthcare procedures on the patient's health. They would include statistics such as surgical mortality rates and/or complications, the rates of successful pregnancies resulting from the various procedures at a fertility clinic, and the percentage of hospitalized patients who are readmitted. While outcome measures seem to be the best quality measure available, results are often skewed by circumstances outside of the healthcare organization's control. **Risk-adjustment methods** can help correct for some factors, but the process is not yet advanced enough to prevent misleading or inaccurate healthcare quality reports.

Healthcare leaders are always aware of comparative data and benchmarking so they are in the best position to identify and select measures for their organization. High volume processes, error prone processes, safety measures and others that are mandated by CMS or a parent organization can result in an organization monitoring several dozen measures each year.

## Developing Scorecards and Dashboards

A **scorecard** is a type of report that measures an organization's performance and compares it against its projections and goals. Modern scorecards are sophisticated software solutions. The scorecard utilizes the organization's data to evaluate the success and failure of **key performance indicators (KPIs)**. If used correctly, scorecards can be an extremely valuable tool. Scorecards allow organizations to assess their current objectives and progress, evaluate trends, and maximize efficient use of resources.

Scorecards started out as a simple framework for measuring performance but have become a robust system for management and strategic planning. Scorecards give performance measurements on daily activities for every part of an organization. Senior management create the vision and strategies which are passed to every part of an organization. These are then used by departments to set objectives and goals, assign responsibilities, and create accountability. Additional training should be given if necessary, in order to help employees meet their department's new goals.

**Dashboards** provide a focused view of summaries, key trends, comparisons, and exceptions. Ideally, a dashboard's design will be simple, have minimal distractions, and provide meaningful data for businesses to make quick and informed decisions. Dashboards are created using multiple reports and make it easy to compare and contrast reports or examine a variety of data sets together. Scorecards may also be used as part of a dashboard to ensure the accuracy of the reports.

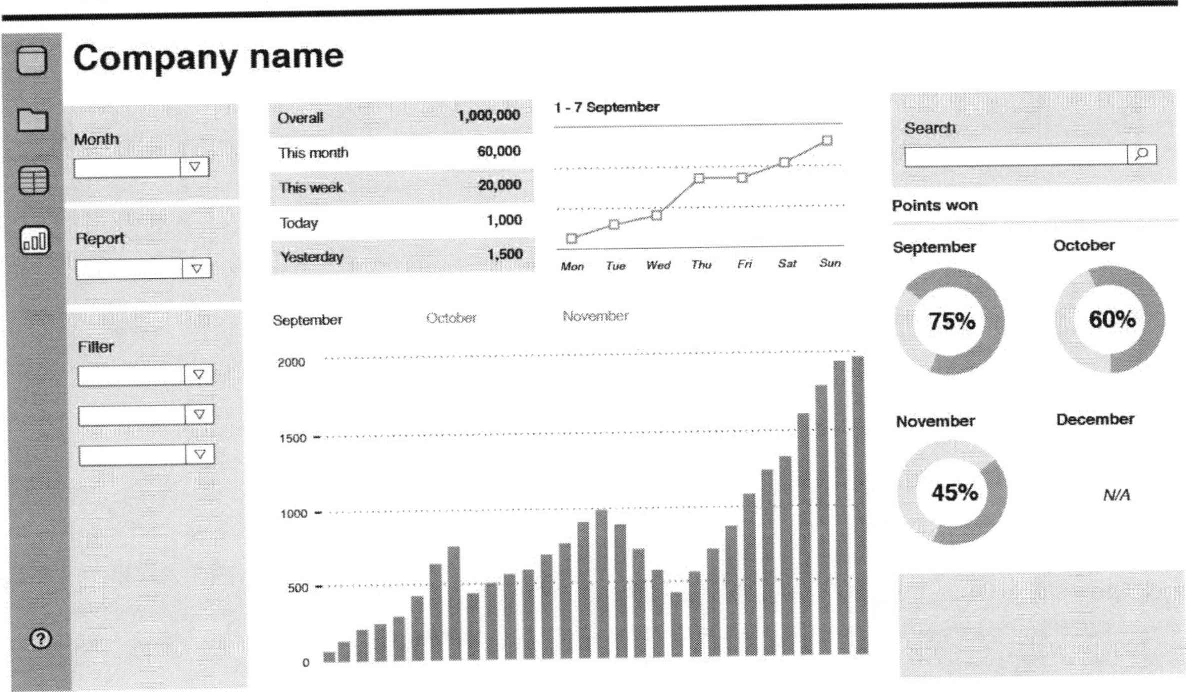


The laws around data are evolving. Privacy is a state of being that every organization must take responsibility for. Each organization must cloak its daily habits using a **VPN (virtual private network)** connection. A VPN service will scramble the signal so that identity and location are at least partially masked from trackers. A VPN will substantially reduce how much the world can observe the organization's online habits. Some of the most common reports used on a dashboard are new item trends, 52-week profit analysis, and exception reports.

## Identifying External Data Sources for Comparison

**Benchmarking** is another method that allows for the analysis of healthcare delivery, trends, and best practices. Benchmarks are useful in that they permit the comparison of apples to apples. This is especially true when audits are internal to an organization. Benchmarking allows the comparison of results with state, regional, or national organizations that are similar in structure. For example, the average length of stay or number of bed days may be a metric that is monitored and even tied to the performance of an organization. Industry benchmarks in managed care organizations include the following:

- Acute-care admissions per thousand
- Acute-care bed days per thousand
- Skilled nursing bed days per thousand
- Home care admissions per thousand
- Home care visits per thousand

The benchmarking exercise can also help to identify processes that have an opportunity for improvement. The exercise supports monitoring of consistency in practice, while also enabling compliance with quality standards. Patients, caregivers, providers, payers, and a variety of other participants in the patient's care should be a part of evaluating their experience. Their feedback is critical in the evaluation of the overall effectiveness of a program.

The leadership team decides which benchmarks are appropriate for their organization and metrics. In most cases the benchmarks are standardized or mandated, as in Joint Commission benchmarks or national quality and patient safety benchmarks. Internal benchmarks are those that the organization determines are important trends to monitor.

## Collecting and Validating Data

When an organization collects its own new data, despite attempts to avoid errors, there can still be mistakes. Because of this, organizations need to validate their data by checking for bad data. When using data from outside sources (e.g., the CDC), it should still be checked after it's been put in the format that the organization intends to use it in. There are a lot of unintentional mistakes that can occur when importing or exporting data, which makes the data validation step one of the most important pieces of data collection and analysis. Data validation should be performed before the data is used in any way by a healthcare organization.

Throughout the data validation process, the leadership team must always be asking whether the results make sense. Common procedures to validate continuous variables include checking the minimum and maximum values, the mean, and the median. For example, when working with hospital data, one of the variables may be how long a patient has lived at their current residence. The first items to check are the minimum and maximum values for how long they've lived at their current address. If the results had a minimum of 0.05 years and a maximum of 47 years, those would be reasonable results. Some patients will have lived at the same location for a long time, while others may have recently moved in. If, instead of those results, the minimum was 50 years and the max was 4.7 years, it would be obvious there's an error in the data. There might have been some mathematical mistakes or data entered incorrectly.

When collecting and validating data, two main checks should be routinely done: confirm whether the data was downloaded correctly, and see if the data was imported into the right format for your analysis software. These are both steps where data mistakes can easily happen. **Cross tabulations**, which display the frequency with which each combination of variables occurs, are often useful when validating data because it allows you to identify combinations that shouldn't occur. For example, when considering a patient's sex and pregnancy status, it's obvious that a male patient should never be listed as pregnant. Regardless of how much effort is made towards creating a good data collection system, there will always

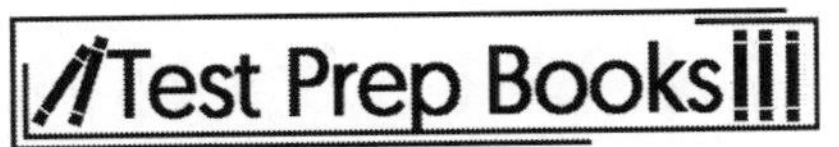

be some errors. These must be fixed during data cleaning, which can be an expensive, complicated, and time-consuming process, but it is necessary for any project that handles data.

# *Measurement and Analysis*

## Data Management Systems

The amount of healthcare data available can seem overwhelming. Healthcare leaders need to drive their organizations to work with a more data-oriented mindset. Administrators and physicians must be diligent when collecting patient data, marketing departments need to utilize data-based outreach, and patients must become more involved in their own healthcare. Everyone in the healthcare industry needs to be involved to make data management a priority.

As the healthcare industry moves aggressively toward outcome-based reimbursement, all healthcare entities need to remodel their operations to focus on affordable, effective and accessible service delivery. Leaders will need to develop strategies to reduce costs and improve collaboration to face the challenges posed by ever-evolving threats to their IT systems and data. It's important to find new ways to efficiently manage people, processes, and technology to deliver integrated and effective care, as well as efficient business services.

The healthcare organization must also be able to adapt to new regulatory requirements and to rationalize and integrate systems in the wake of mergers and acquisitions or consolidation of payers and providers. Strategic thinking about the application of new technology is crucial to improving IT cost efficiency and quality. Without a strategic approach, organizations might inadvertently put money into technology that doesn't integrate well with their business or increase its value.

**Healthcare data management** involves storing, protecting, and analyzing data gathered from multiple sources. Providers need to be able to manage all their available data to develop comprehensive views of patients, individualize patient care, enhance communication, and improve outcomes. There are thousands of different data management systems and each organization must fit their IT needs into both the fiscal plan and the operational plan each year. Senior leaders and IT management must work together to determine which products best meet the needs of the organization. A few of the data management systems include the following:

### Electronic Health Record (EHR):

**Electronic Health Records (EHRs)** allow physicians and other medical personnel to simplify the medical recording process by electronically recording and storing patient information. By using EHRs, hospitals and other organizations can securely access and consolidate patients' medical records. The EHR replaces the paper medical charts and contains everything from physician orders and lab work to surgical notes and medications. Each patient has a specific record with unique identifiers.

### Healthcare Customer Relations Management (HCRM):

**Healthcare Customer Relations Management (HCRM)** systems are able to integrate, measure, analyze, and report on data from multiple sources, all inside one data hub. This technology enables organizations to consolidate consumer and patient data from EHRs and other sources, such as engagement centers and social media. By utilizing healthcare CRM technology, organizations can gain a comprehensive view of patients that covers the patient lifecycle as well as consumer profiles, preferences, and behaviors.

### Reliability Centered Maintenance (RCM)

**Reliability Centered Maintenance (RCM)** is typically used to create improvements such as the establishment of safe minimum levels of maintenance. Successfully implementing RCM will improve cost effectiveness, improve machine uptime, improve reliability, and give a better understanding of the risk the organization manages. RCM helps businesses create cost-effective maintenance plans that deal with the causes of equipment failure. This process finds the main function of routinely maintained equipment and determines the primary modes, causes, and consequences of failure, and then identifies the criticality level of each of those consequences. RCM focuses on addressing failures that can be solved with preventative maintenance before they ever happen. However, some functions that are less important are allowed to continue until a failure occurs, whereas highly critical functions are maintained to prevent any risk of failure. When there is a high risk associated with a function, RCM may recommend or require changing something to lower the risk. This system enables the organization increase cost-effectiveness by pre-emptively focusing on processes with the most harmful consequences of failure.

### Enterprise Application Software (EAS)

**Enterprise Application Software (EAS)** is used to address the needs of an organization as a whole, as opposed to the needs of individuals. These organizations may include charities, education systems, businesses, or government. Because businesses frequently have overlapping divisions and processes, enterprise software is often customizable, in order to address issues that affect an entire organization rather than specific departments. The goal of EAS is to increase productivity by providing tools that utilize business logic. This software is usually hosted on servers and allows many users across a network to access its services at the same time. The services that EAS provides are usually business tools, such as the following:

- Online payment processing
- Security systems
- Human resource management
- Occupational health and safety
- Project management
- IT service management
- Customer relationship management
- Business intelligence

## Using Tools to Display Data or Evaluate a Process

The most effective format for the dissemination and depiction of statistical data is often via a graph or chart. For those not familiar with data interpretation, visual tools such as Pareto charts, run charts, scattergrams, and control charts can easily depict the trends and correlational relationships between variables. Leadership teams will utilize appropriate tools to display data related to the organization's mission, values, and goals.

A **Pareto chart** depicts data in the form of bars placed in descending order, with a line representing the cumulative total. The 80-20 rule, otherwise known as the Pareto principle, states that for a given event, nearly 80% of effects can be attributed to 20% of causes. This rule is frequently used in business to highlight that the majority of revenue comes from roughly one fifth of its clientele. Consequently, the Pareto principle is used for identifying which items have the largest effect on the business and allow management to focus on the important factors in a cost-efficient manner.

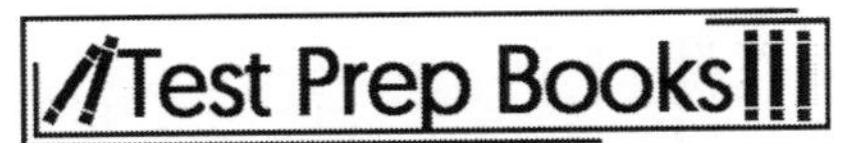

Supplementary quality control tools include the run chart, control charts, histograms, scatter plot diagrams, and check sheets. Both the **run** and the **control charts** are line graphs that depict data points along a continuum; however, the control chart includes a control limit. Both charts also clearly indicate trends and patterns of specific processes and how well that process is performing. While control charts are best utilized when monitoring processes on an ongoing basis, run charts are best suited for investigating short-term process improvement activities.

**Histograms** graphically represent the variation of values within a group. This format depicts the center, spread, and shape of the data. The distribution will be distinctly normal, bi-modal, or skewed. One final format for depicting statistical data is the **fishbone**, or **cause and effect diagram**. Named for the shape, this diagram focuses largely on depicting the precipitating factors, or root causes, for a specific event or outcome. Those root causes can be separated into more meaningful categories. Practitioners can then engage in the brainstorming necessary to clarify potential solutions. This format for representing data is also useful when there is little quantitative data accessible for analysis.

Although every program and process evaluation project does not require the use of each tool, at least two charts are typically utilized for precision when reporting results.

## Using Statistics to Describe Data

Historically, statisticians utilize measures of central tendency when evaluating any set of data. The three most common measures of central tendency include the mean, median, and mode. The **mean** is the average of the sample and is determined by adding all of the outcomes from the sample then dividing it by the total number of events. The **median** is the middle value within the data set when all results are presented in ascending or descending order. If the midpoint consists of two numbers, then the average is to be taken of the two. The **mode** is the most common value appearing within the data set. The **range** is the difference in the span of values within the complete set, or the largest value minus the smallest value. When a normal data set is generated, the data are depicted as a bell-shaped curve; the mean, median, and mode are the same.

**Variance** is the sum of the squared deviations from the mean, divided by the total size of the sample. The standard deviation is defined as the average distance of all points of data from the mean of the data set. The correlation, or dependent relationship between two quantitative continuous variables, can either be positive or negative. For example, if one variable increases corresponding to the increase of another, the two variables are said to be positively correlated. Alternatively, if one variable decreases while another increases, that relationship is considered to be negatively correlated. One additional measure, a **t-test**, is used to compare the differences between the means of separate distributions. The t-test is a statistical tool that usually is done in Minitab or a similar software. It is generally thought to guide the determination of root causality between two processes.

## Statistical Process Control

**Statistical Process Control (SPC)** is a standard method of measuring and maintaining quality that has long been used in manufacturing. Product (outcome) and process measures are collected in real time during manufacturing and used as quality data to develop control charts to track causes of variation. This method is similarly useful in healthcare quality control. The control chart's upper and lower limits are determined by a process's capabilities, and specification limits may be set according to regulations. Data is expected to be within the control limits, and variations inside this range are mostly due to common causes. Data that goes outside of the control limits often indicates a special cause that can be identified as the reason for the variations, and changes can then be made to prevent the issue from recurring. SPC can significantly improve outcomes and productivity, reduce variability and costs, and it allows leaders to quickly react to process changes.

SPC has been a manufacturing standard for decades but it is only within the past 20 years that it has been used in healthcare. The thinking is that an error is an error and waste is waste, whether the process is patient-related or material-related. The process is what is important to control in order to reduce costs and eliminate rework.

**Common cause variation**, also called **random variation**, is the process by which numerous small general factors result in a specific effect on a process. These stressors to the process are predictable and occur in every process. For example, consider the effect of staffing in a typical emergency room. If it is determined that there is a thirty-minute wait for patients to be examined by a physician once admitted to an emergency room, the management can simply act to permanently increase staffing to the ER; or reduce the possibility of variance.

**Special cause variation** refers to the specific rare factors that can influence a process. These are new and unexpected stressors that occur sporadically. Considering the same example, special cause variation in this instance would be a wait of three hours for a patient to be examined once admitted to the ER. Upon further examination, the evaluator may uncover a specific event of staff being preoccupied caring for numerous patients involved in a local apartment building fire. The best way to solve this problem would be to institute disaster protocols, whereby specific individuals throughout the facility can be dispatched to the ER to manage the overflow when it does occur. Both interventions would require approaching the problem at its roots, engaging in corrective or preventative actions, and mitigating as much variation as possible.

A **trend analysis** is a method based on historical data about a process. There are no fully automatic methods that can identify trends in time series, but if there is a consistent increase or decrease in the data, the trend might be obvious. If the data contains significant noise or errors, the first step to find a trend will be smoothing. **Smoothing** takes the average, or mean, of data inside a limited range so irregularities will equal out. It's also possible to use the median values instead of means to smooth data. One significant advantage to using medians it that outliers will have less effect on the data being smoothed, giving more reliable results.

The majority of patterns seen in time series data are describable by their trend and seasonality. **Trend** is defined as the general, systematic, linear or nonlinear changes in a component over time, which doesn't repeat during the time bring observed. **Seasonality**, on the other hand, is the repetitiveness in a data set. For example, over several years, a business may experience a significant overall rise in sales, but still have seasonal patterns of increasing and decreasing sales over each month, season, or year.

## Interpreting Data to Support Decision-Making

Once the leadership team has gathered, analyzed, and discussed the aggregated data, they will create a dialogue that will lead to the necessary changes. As the team interprets the data, they must keep in mind that a hypothesis cannot be proven true; one can only fail to reject the hypothesis. This means

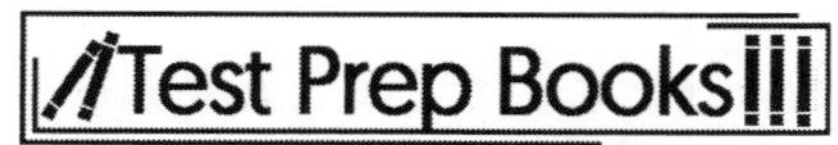

that no matter how much data the team collects, chance can always interfere with the results. Therefore, when interpreting the results of data, the leadership team must ask the following questions:

- Does the data answer our original question? How?
- Does the data help defend against any objections? How?
- Are there any limitations on our conclusions; any angles we haven't considered?

If the interpretation of the data can stand rigorous enough questioning, then the team has likely produced a useful conclusion. All that remains is to utilize the data analysis results to develop an action plan. As team members gain familiarity with data analysis, the process becomes faster and more accurate, and the organization will run more effectively by using well-informed decisions.

## Comparing Data Sources to Establish Benchmarks

The cornerstone of data management is to ensure that the organization is reaching pre-determined goals. **Benchmarking** in healthcare is essentially the process of comparing one healthcare organization's performance against that of other organizations. A more technical definition is that benchmarking is a process in which the results of fundamental healthcare processes are continually measured and compared. Typically, the ideas and practices of the best performers are compared with the host organization. The four distinct types of benchmarking for quality improvement include:

- Internal: comparing equivalent processes within the same organization
- Competitive: comparing similar processes to a competitor within the same industry
- Functional: comparing similar processes to those in different industries
- Generic: comparing the general concepts of processes in unrelated industries

Staff progress can be measured internally, and the separate business functions can be compared externally. Leadership within the organization can employ comparative analysis on a cyclical, weekly, or daily basis in an effort to respond to concerns in real time, rather than after the impact has reached the consumer.

It will be necessary to have frequent brainstorming sessions. **Brainstorming** can be referred to as a way of using a selected group of individuals to rapidly produce, clarify, and evaluate ideas or problems. Staff must be encouraged to preview the preliminary data, and leadership must allow for an open-ended and honest critique of what does and does not work. It is important to note that there are no right or wrong answers in brainstorming sessions, as the object is to generate momentum around finding solutions by coming up with as many ideas as possible. Brainstorming offers the team an opportunity to view all aspects of the problem and can often yield unexpected results. Results shared within the organization help each employee to connect with the results and recognize that they can affect change through their individual behaviors.

Internal benchmarking efforts encourage top performers to form more practical solutions to problems articulated by the data. Competitive benchmarking can help delineate how similar organizations solved similar defects. The comparative analysis can also reveal how the current processes are outpacing the competitors, which encourages the integration of what works with what does not work well enough. This approach will help the leadership team to deliver on the promise of providing exceptional care.

## Participating in External Reporting

Once the leadership team has established the overall mission and goals of the healthcare organization, the next step will be to ensure that quality and safety activities are in alignment with those goals. Data gleaned from the internal and competitive benchmarking and brainstorming sessions are meant to transform processes and procedures that have no statistically significant value added to the business. Aggregated data must be analyzed to reveal trends in the data that indicate which of the organizations' established goals and objectives can be translated into critical success factors. These are then used to create KPI—measurable data that will further indicate if the goals and objectives are attainable. The data or input measures are typically representative of services or skill level, whereas output measures represent outcomes and results.

The **Healthcare Effectiveness Data and Information Set (HEDIS)** is a group of performance standards that the majority of health plans adhere to in an effort to standardize the overall quality of care delivered to patients. These standards include areas related to quality of care, access to care, and member satisfaction. In its entirety, HEDIS comprises a total of 92 diverse measures across six specific types of care. This data information set allows for equanimity among organizations and health plans and creates a more competitive approach to meeting the numerous quality standards among healthcare systems. Health plans can utilize the reported results to gauge their performance against those reported by competitors. This comparison tool is a registered and trademarked strategy of the **National Committee for Quality Assurance (NCQA)**. This data clearinghouse allows for an internal benchmark, as health plans can review their own previous results and identify upward and downward trends. The **Quality Compass** is an interactive web-based tool within the NCQA arsenal that generates quality reports based on specific plans, benchmarks, and time frames.

One additional facet of the HEDIS quality standards is the **Consumer Assessment of Healthcare Providers and Systems (CAHPS)** survey, which was developed in 1995 as a method for quantifying members' satisfaction regarding their overall experience with specific health plans. The general public had previously struggled to locate information regarding the standards of quality achieved and the members' subsequent satisfaction. The NCQA encourages the exchange of quality information to consumers who can view both quality adherence statistics and accreditation standards. By viewing the State of Health Care Quality report, consumers are better equipped to monitor the report cards of healthcare plans and organizations. Completed annually, the primary goal of this quality report is focused improvement of the dissemination, implementation, and spread of evidence-based care across the country.

CMS, commercial health plans, and private physicians, as well as healthcare leaders and legislators, worked diligently to develop the Core Quality Measure Collaborative. The **Core Quality Measures** were developed to promote evidence-based care, decrease healthcare expenditures, and encourage providers to utilize bundling of services.

**Bundled payments**, also known as **episode of care payment** or **package pricing**, can be defined as a single payment made to cover the costs of the treatment provided for any given service. Led by the **America's Health Insurance Plans (AHIP)**, this initiative was established to encourage payers to employ a set of core measures to utilize during reporting. The Core Measures include the following: Cardiology, Gastroenterology, HIV and Hepatitis C, Medical Oncology, Obstetrics and Gynecology, Orthopedics, Pediatrics, Accountable Care Organizations, Patient Centered Medical Homes, and Primary Care. It is

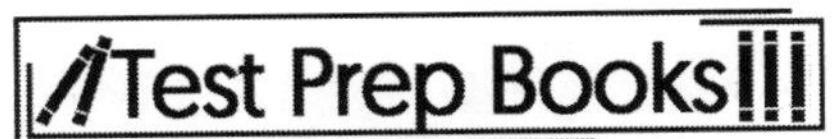

important to note that the primary purpose of reporting significant findings is the adherence to specific standards of excellence.

## Practice Quiz

1. What diagram is used to brainstorm all possible causes of a problem in order to sort ideas into categories that ultimately lead to a solution?
    a. Plan-Do-Check-Act (PDCA) cycle
    b. Fishbone diagram
    c. Quality planning road map
    d. Value stream map

2. Which of the following statements is true about random sampling?
    a. There is a less than equal probability of all units being selected when utilizing random sampling methods.
    b. This method requires extensive information about the population being sampled.
    c. This method can be used when little information is provided about the population being sampled.
    d. None of the above

3. Which measure for the center of a small sample set would be most affected by outliers?
    a. Mean
    b. Median
    c. Mode
    d. None of the above

4. Estimation and hypothesis testing are the two main types of which of the following?
    a. Descriptive statistics
    b. Statistical distributions
    c. Inferential statistics
    d. None of the above

5. A box-and- whisker plot of yearly salaries for car salespersons has a Q 1 of $45,000, Q 2 of $51,000, and a Q 3 of $59,000. Which of the following salaries would be considered outliers for the set?

    I. $21,000
    II. $28,000
    III. $65,000
    IV. $85,000

    a. I only
    b. IV only
    c. I and IV
    d. I, II, III, and IV

**See answers on next page.**

## Answer Explanations

**1. B:** The fishbone diagram is used to brainstorm all possible causes of a problem so that ideas can be sorted into categories that ultimately lead to a solution. The Plan-Do-Check-Act (PDCA) cycle is an ongoing evaluation of procedures and managerial policies leading to continuous improvement, and it is made up of four stages. The quality planning road map provides a more detailed approach to the activities associated with each of the three processes within Dr. Joseph M. Juran's Trilogy. Finally, a value stream map is a visual means to identify and analyze a specific business process within a company.

**2. C:** Random sampling entails randomly drawing an item so that every item drawn has an equal chance of being included in the sample. In other words, there is an equal probability with random sampling. Random sampling is a fairly simple and cost-effective method often used when little information can be obtained about the items in the population.

**3. A:** Mean. An outlier is a data value that's either far above or below the majority of values in a sample set. The mean is the average of all values in the set. In a small sample, a very high or low number could greatly change the average. The median is the middle value when arranged from lowest to highest. Outliers would have no more of an effect on the median than any other value. Mode is the value that repeats most often in a set. Assuming that the same outlier doesn't repeat, outliers would have no effect on the mode of a sample set.

**4. C:** Inferential statistics. Estimation and hypothesis testing are the two main types of inferential statistics, which are used to analyze the strength of the relationship between independent and dependent variables.

**5. C:** I and IV. Outliers in a box-and-whisker plot are data points that fall below the lower extreme or above the upper extreme. The lower extreme is calculated by subtracting 1.5 times the interquartile range from $Q_1$. And the upper extreme is calculated by adding 1.5 times the interquartile range to $Q_3$. In this case, the interquartile range ($Q_3$-$Q_1$) is 14,000. Therefore, the lower extreme is $24,000 and the upper extreme is $80,000.

## Identifying Opportunities for Improvement

### Facilitating Discussion About Quality Improvement Opportunities

A facilitator plans, guides, and manages group events to make sure that the meeting's objectives are reached and that all members become involved, clearly express their thoughts, and agree on a solution. A good facilitator needs to be objective; they must take a neutral stance on the topics discussed and instead focus on managing the group process.

The first step to a successful meeting is defining what the meeting should achieve. This ought to be done even before sending out meeting invitations, because determining a clear objective will help delineate who will need to be present at the meeting, how long the meeting should last, and what should be on the meeting's agenda. The facilitator should also pause before sending a meeting invite to evaluate whether or not a meeting is the best means to achieve the stated objective or if they should pursue a different technique (e.g., observation, workshops, interviews, etc.). Finally, knowing and articulating the desired outcome of a meeting sets expectations for the meeting and can also be used to measure the success of the meeting and any outcomes resulting from the meeting. If the outcomes achieve the stated goal, then the meeting and its subsequent effects were a success.

The facilitator should limit the group to a number between 5 and 20 people. This will ensure that the facilitator will only select participants who are actually necessary for the meeting, while also being respectful of stakeholders' time. Persons who have expressed an interest in the topic, people with power, and people with knowledge of the task at hand are all good choices for team members.

Preparation for meetings is essential. The facilitator should have a clear and concise agenda, get the information out well in advance of the meeting, and it may be necessary to personally brief attendees. If there is a possibility of conflict, the facilitator must understand why in advance and have a plan to deescalate any conflict.

The facilitator must assign a scribe who can also help with any logistical items. Ensure that the meeting room is booked and large enough, equipment (projector, flip-charts, slides) is available and working, and that the facilitator has notes and anything else needed for the meeting.

**Group process** is the method used to of manage group discussion, receive input from all participants, and have the event arrive at a successful conclusion. Optimal facilitation enables the group to generate ideas, solutions, and decisions. To do this, facilitators design the group process and provide tools that will help the group arrive at that outcome. The facilitator is responsible for guiding the group process to achieve a productive outcome. Ideally, there must be strong participation among group members, they must arrive at a consensus, everyone's input should be acknowledged and used in developing ideas, solutions, and decisions, and all participants should share responsibility for the results.

The facilitator must also make sure that all questions, actions, and outcomes are documented and properly handled. The task of recording group process may also be delegated to a scribe, to free up the facilitator to more easily handle other tasks during the event. The following items must be considered when facilitating a group event:

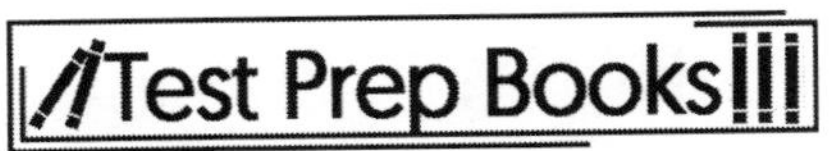

- Whether there should be open discussion or a structured process
- If variety of topics needed can be covered
- Whether enough ideas and solutions can be generated
- The facilitator's own ability to get everyone's involvement and buy-in
- The number of participants
- The nature of the topics being discussed
- The type of involvement needed
- The background and positions of the participants
- How well the participants understand the subject and other members
- The time available

There are many organizational devices that a facilitator can use to help the meeting run smoothly:

- Ice Breakers, to ease group contributions
- Multivoting, for choosing fairly between multiple options
- Brainstorming, for producing many ideas
- Role Playing, to prepare for difficult situations
- Small group discussion
- Paired listening
- Eisenhower matrix (Urgent/important grid)
- Pros and cons list
- Plus-Minus-Implications list

The last step in preparing for group events is to consider how the meeting will be run and organized. It's beneficial to set ground rules for the event so that the meeting stays under control, people respect each other's ideas, and that questions are handled appropriately. The facilitator should also plan some ground rules ahead of time to present at the start of the meeting. To ensure the meeting runs smoothly, there are several things an effective facilitator should do:

- Set the scene. Give participants an overview of the meeting, including the agenda and objectives. Ensure that everyone knows their role and the purpose of the event.

- Get things flowing. Have all participants introduce themselves and use icebreakers to positively kickstart the event.

- Keep up the momentum and energy. Intercede as the event progresses and energy levels change. Keep participants attentive and focused on the discussion.

- Listen, engage, and include. Set a positive example for participants by staying alert, actively listening, and staying engaged and interested. This also enables the facilitator to intervene if needed.

- Monitor checkpoints and summarize. Stay on top of schedule, let participants know what's been covered, and tell them what will happen next. Frequently summarize the event, and only intervene if necessary.

- Record, aggregate, and address actionable output. The facilitator is responsible for making sure the ideas, solutions, and outcomes from the event are recorded. They should gather the event's output and share it with the group, and will need to ensure that action is taken from event outcomes.

- Refresh the group on the discussion thus far, maintain group focus, and keep progressing towards the objectives. If the facilitator is unsure that the recordkeeping is accurate to the discussion, they should get clarification before moving on.
- Provide follow-up after the meeting to make sure that actionable items are addressed, and that the proceedings arrive at a successful conclusion.

A good agenda may only have a few action items. It is better to focus on broad objectives first and drill down to more specific objectives. As an example:

- Brainstorm session: What worked well this year and what didn't? (15 min)
- Determine priority items down to top five (10 min)
- Action plans for the top 3 (20 min)
- Questions/concerns/next steps (10 min)

The final step in a successful meeting is follow-up. Without clear action items, delegation, and dates for implementation and review, even the best meeting will have no lasting effect. Making sure that these items are in place before a meeting ends will help ensure useful and complete follow-up.

When a decision is made to initiate a performance or process improvement project, healthcare organizations typically begin by reviewing all areas of weakness. Primarily, those areas are determined by reviewing the business goals, mission, vision, and values of the organization, along with the associated **key performance indicators (KPIs)**. The basic framework of the project is built on this needs assessment. It is also necessary to determine the **critical to quality measures (CTQs)**, which are the aspects of a business process or product that must be met in order to satisfy the consumer. Once a significant list has been compiled, the team can begin to define the problem.

Ideally, organizations seeking to maintain a high level of excellence should consider evaluating the internal **voice of the business (VOB)**. The VOB reflects the specific needs and concerns of the healthcare organization as a business and may include concerns such as profit, growth, and competitiveness. When designing an appropriate process flow for a client-centered service, it will be crucial to determine the must have aspects of that service according to the customer, or the **voice of the customer (VOC)**. The consumer's voice is the outward image of the business and the reputation that the business has earned among consumers. Building on the external VOC and the internal VOB, the project management team must work collaboratively to ensure that performance and production waste are eliminated, while simultaneously improving overall organizational efficiency and revenue. When standards and policies that were originally created to satisfy the customer according to the CTQs are not consistently met, the business begins to falter. It is important to ascertain whether the projected business goals meet or exceed the VOC and VOB, or whether they have conflicting interests.

When the business's needs do not match the customer's needs, resources can become exhausted. The team will conduct a needs assessment based on the priority of CTQs to calculate how projected goals from previous quarters differ from current results. These needs assessments are performed throughout the company and on all crucial processes and procedures. Specialized departments that handle more intricate issues may have a more stringent process and procedure assessment schedule. Apparent gaps in outcomes related to the VOC and the VOB must be addressed and the staff retrained in an effort to

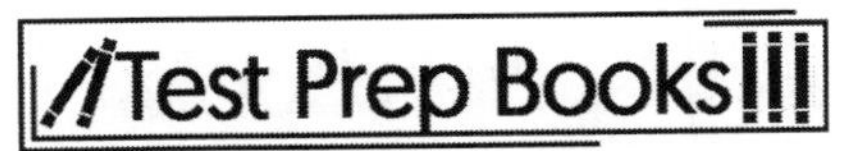

standardize policies, procedures, and processes. Addressing CTQs enables the project management team to focus on the problem.

## Establishing Priorities

Each healthcare organization must prioritize monitoring various aspects of care according to its unique situation and types of care provided. The focus should be on the areas of care that are provided most frequently, those which are considered high risk, and any areas of care that are particularly problematic for the given organization. Screening methodologies and peer review can both help organizations pinpoint where their priorities should be and avoid wasting resources attempting to monitor all aspects of care all the time. An organization's leadership must also ensure that their teams are up to date on the best definitions of high-quality care and are committed to constant improvement by utilizing review programs that are continuous, priority-oriented, and effective. The 80/20 rule must also be acknowledged and investigated. All indicators and criteria used to monitor care must be consistent with current state-of-the-art practice. Leaders must invest time and funds to improving diffusion of current clinical knowledge to practitioners. They must be equally aware that substandard care may occur and seek new ways to improve that care.

Establishing priorities for monitoring aspects of care is particularly important in light of the numerous efforts to control healthcare costs and the effect of those cost-control measures on healthcare quality. Consumers are increasingly interested in quality comparisons between healthcare plans and healthcare providers, and are also becoming more aware of the aspects of care that are most important to their individual situations.

One effect of this growing consumer-orientation in healthcare is that care is increasingly provided outside of hospitals and other inpatient settings. The quality of care in settings such as ambulatory care, home care, rehabilitation centers, specialized outpatient service centers, etc. directly impacts the ability of hospitals to provide quality inpatient care, and the quality of inpatient care also affects the ability of providers in other settings to provide quality care. Providers in all healthcare settings must coordinate their efforts and track patient care across an illness or episode of care to track and improve quality outcomes rather than focusing on the quality of one setting alone. Quality evaluation is a critically important element of healthcare service and must be a priority for staff at every level of all healthcare organizations.

Despite best efforts, mistakes and issues can and will occur in healthcare settings. These events must be carefully evaluated and continuously monitored in order to devise processes that will eliminate, or at least minimize, such events and improve care. Various methodologies are available to assist healthcare organizations in identifying areas that need the most improvement in quality of care. For example, a **Pareto analysis** could be used to illustrate how a relatively small number of areas account for majority of variation. By finding the most costly departments, there are areas that can be focused on. This provides healthcare organizations a starting point for improving quality, beginning with the processes that have the largest variation in quality. Setting and agreeing upon priorities allows healthcare providers to efficiently reduce variations and improve care.

## Facilitating Development of Action Plans or Projects

An action plan should be more than just a list of what activities to carry out. An ideal action plan should answer some basic questions by including the following items:

- A time frame (When will it happen?)
- Assessment of the existing capacities, to identify missing capacities (How will it be done?)
- A cost evaluation (How much will it cost?)
- Identification of the actors (Who will take part?)
- Appropriate mechanisms to track and evaluate progress (Why/What for?)

In other words, an action plan should answer the five W's and one H: who, what, when, where, why, and how.

Each objective in an action plan needs to have a clear purpose and well-defined outputs. The action plan should be used in a logical framework, which shows the interventions taken to develop statistics. The framework consists of a few components:

- Overall objective: The broad development impact brought about in part by the project
- Outcome: The development outcome after the strategy's implementation, especially the predicted benefits for target groups
- Outputs: The direct and tangible results to be delivered, which are largely controlled by project management
- Activities: The actions that must be performed to produce the expected results
- Indicators: Connected to the objective-oriented planning and measure how the objectives, purpose, results, and activities will be accomplished

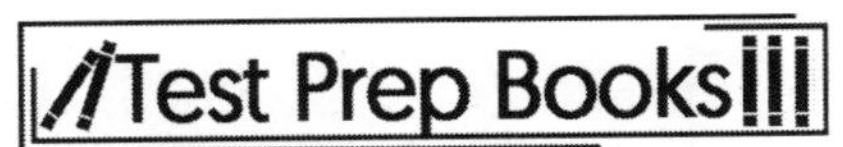


An action plan should be well-defined and used daily by the team leader to manage the actions, expenses, and timeline of a project. Additionally, it should be used in monitoring and evaluating the project's strategic implementation, making adjustments as needed, and assessing the results.

### Example of an Action Plan

| Goal 1 | Action Step Descriptions | Party/Dept Responsible | Date to begin | Date due |
|---|---|---|---|---|
| *Write your goal statement here* | | | | |
| *List resources and desired outcomes* | | | | |

| Goal 2 | Action Step Descriptions | Party/Dept Responsible | Date to begin | Date due |
|---|---|---|---|---|
| *Write your goal statement here* | | | | |
| *List resources and desired outcomes* | | | | |

| Goal 3 | Action Step Descriptions | Party/Dept Responsible | Date to begin | Date due |
|---|---|---|---|---|
| *Write your goal statement here* | | | | |
| *List resources and desired outcomes* | | | | |

| Goal 4 | Action Step Descriptions | Party/Dept Responsible | Date to begin | Date due |
|---|---|---|---|---|
| *Write your goal statement here* | | | | |
| *List resources and desired outcomes* | | | | |

## Performance Improvement Methods

As mentioned earlier, there are four terms that apply to starting a new process or method in an organization:

- **Diffusion** occurs when new practices spread passively, without deliberate implementation.

- **Dissemination** occurs when new practices are deliberately implemented and actively spread. Plans for dissemination usually identify a target audience and outline specific methodologies.
- **Implementation** occurs when those practices are adopted and integrated within a healthcare setting.
- **Spread** refers to the rate at which newly disseminated ideas or innovations are adopted and implemented.

One key principle is that quality insurance cannot be a one-and-done effort. No matter how good and thorough the implemented methodologies are, healthcare processes must be continuously evaluated and improved in order to continue to provide quality of care. Lessons learned can be used to shift strategy and try new interventions.

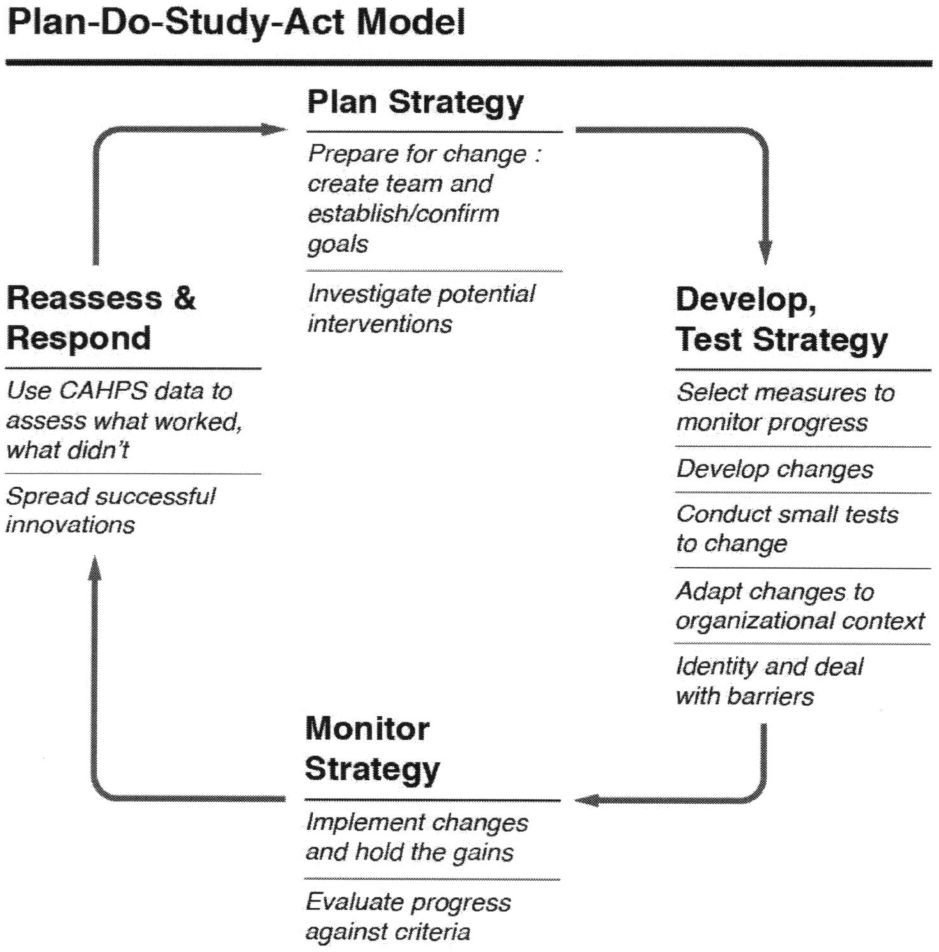

**Plan-Do-Study-Act Model**

**Plan Strategy**

*Prepare for change : create team and establish/confirm goals*

*Investigate potential interventions*

**Develop, Test Strategy**

*Select measures to monitor progress*

*Develop changes*

*Conduct small tests to change*

*Adapt changes to organizational context*

*Identity and deal with barriers*

**Monitor Strategy**

*Implement changes and hold the gains*

*Evaluate progress against criteria*

**Reassess & Respond**

*Use CAHPS data to assess what worked, what didn't*

*Spread successful innovations*

## PDSA

One of the most useful healthcare improvement models is the PDSA cycle, illustrated in the figure above. PDSA stans for Plan, Do, Study, Act – the four fundamental elements of any improvement plan or methodology. These four steps lay out a continuous cycle of evaluation and improvement, based on the idea that all elements of a healthcare system are interdependent, and even small changes in one area

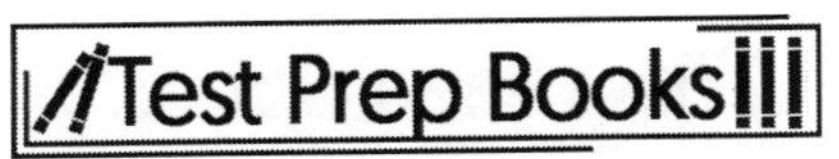

can have large effects across the system. The PDSA cycle provides a straightforward methodology that involves staff at every level of a healthcare organization in the process of discovering problems, coming up with solutions, and then testing the new systems. Because it involves the providers who use the healthcare systems on a daily basis as well as the organization's leadership, this model provides the greatest likelihood for systemic, continuous, and successful improvement in quality care.

The four parts of the PDSA model are explained below.

### *Plan*

The first step in the PDSA cycle focuses on defining goals, developing a strategy, and determining the measurements for success. When using PDSA to improve a healthcare process, the first step is to identify possible goals and strategies to implement. Each goal must be specific, measurable, and feasible. Having the goal clearly articulated will support communication across the healthcare organization and will ensure that each staff member knows the objective.

The second part of the Plan step is to develop a strategy that seem likely to achieve the stated objective. This strategy must consider potential barriers to implementation as well as the likelihood of achieving the stated goal. For example, are there any cultural issues or organizational compatibility issues that will make a given strategy difficult to implement? The strategy must also be streamlined to directly suit the specific problem being addressed. Utilizing input from staff, patients, and members is a good way to achieve this portion of the Plan step.

The third part of the Plan step is to lay out the measurements that will determine whether or not the strategy was successful. It is vitally important to pay attention to the desired outcome and make sure that the success metrics will actually measure whether or not that outcome has been achieved. Tools such as control and run charts, dashboard reports, and tables of aggregated data are all means by which the success metrics can be presented and assessed.

### *Do*

The second step of the PDSA cycle is where the plan is implemented. This involves preparing a written action plan for the healthcare organization that states the goals and strategies developed in the Plan step. It should also include specific action items necessary for the implementation of the strategies and a calendar that ensures various actions are completed in the correct order and that the overall timeline is feasible. Utilizing the Gantt chart format is extremely helpful at this stage. It is also important during this step to ensure that the measures to be taken directly address the key elements of the improvements that the organization wishes to make. There should not be so many measures that they overwhelm the organization's staff, but there should not be so few measures that the organization does not have sufficient information to track the success of the changes made.

### *Study*

The third step of the PDSA cycle is where the results of the plan are measured to see if they are successful or if there are additional issues and areas that need improvement. Small-scale testing is particularly useful at this point because it allows for corrections in smaller teams or areas before a plan is implemented more broadly. It is also easier to implement incremental modifications to a plan in a smaller area rather than throughout the organization as a whole; with small-scale testing, every element of the plan is more responsive to change and can be more easily measured, and if a plan does not work it the failure will not be organization wide. The primary element in this step is to study and review the results of the small-scale testing and adjust the plan as necessary to achieve the stated goals. Once the small-scale testing is a success, the plan can more easily be implemented across the entire organization. An additional benefit of achieving success with small-scale testing before wider implementation is that enthusiasm and positive word-of-mouth acknowledge early successes, which will most likely encourage participation and engagement across the organization when it is time for wider implementation.

### *Act*

The fourth step of the PDSA cycle brings the cycle full circle by evaluating what has been learned throughout the process and using it to adapt and alter the goals, methodologies, action items, etc., or, if necessary, go back to the drawing board and revise the current initiative or compose a new initiative altogether. Implementation is expanded to reach sustainable improvement. While all of the other steps are necessary, the Act step of the PDSA cycle is the most important element of ensuring continuous improvement and is the area where healthcare organizations focus the majority of their time.

The PDSA cycle is a flexible methodology that can be customized to fit the needs of any organization. There is no set length of time that a cycle must take; instead, that is left up to the particular organization. Additionally, while are no rules for frequency of monitoring, most organizations choose to monitor either monthly or quarterly.

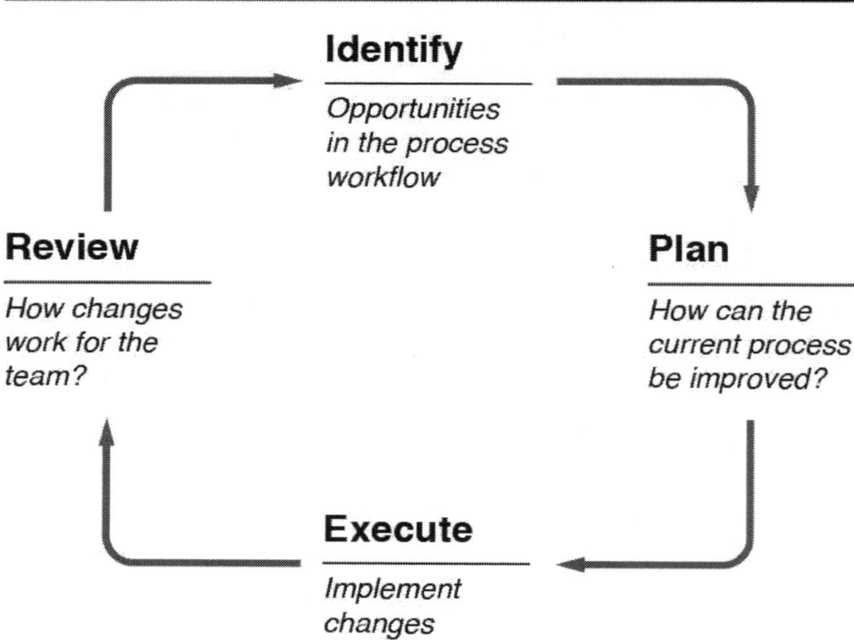

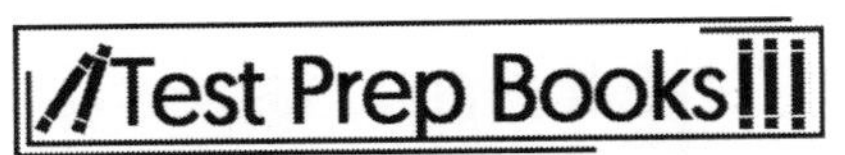

## Six Sigma and Lean

**Lean Six Sigma** is a fact- and data-based quality improvement philosophy that prioritizes the prevention of events over detection. The method improves customer satisfaction and the bottom-line by reducing or eliminating process variations, inefficiencies, and cycle time. Additionally, it encourages the use of workflow standardization to gain a competitive business advantage. Every employee should be involved in Lean Six Sigma because it can be applied to any process where variations or waste are found. The Six Sigma methodology treats all forms of work as processes that are able to be defined, measured, analyzed, improved, and controlled. Processes can be described in terms of their inputs ($x$) and outputs ($y$), and if their inputs are controlled, the outputs will be as well. This allows a process to be quantified and expressed mathematically as $y = f(x)$.

Continued progress in the field of quality improvement has blurred the line between Six Sigma and Lean. The term "Lean Six Sigma" is being used with increasing frequency because both Six Sigma and Lean offer benefits in process improvement. The Six Sigma philosophy is focused on eliminating variations and improving control in processes; it achieves these goals through quantitative methods including statistical data analysis and the process of designing and testing experiments and hypotheses. Lean, on the other hand, is focused on removing waste and inefficiencies and promoting work standardization and flow; it achieves these goals through continuous quality improvement, visual controls, and organization. Both process improvement philosophies aim to provide customers with the best quality, value, delivery, and nimbleness.

Lean has been used by top organizations to maximize their efficiency and effectiveness, reduce waste, and map value streams to gain enhanced understanding of their throughput. Organizations using Six Sigma assign teams to handle clearly-defined projects that will directly benefit their bottom line. Training in statistical thinking is provided to all levels of the organization and key individuals are given further training in advanced statistics and project management. Practitioners of the Lean Six Sigma approach must participate in a series of certification levels, known as belts. Each level signifies the practitioner's knowledge, training, and expertise. A Master Black Belt coaches black belts and green belts. A Black Belt coaches project teams and leads problem-solving projects. A Green Belt helps with data collection and analysis for Black Belt projects and leads Green Belt projects. The Yellow Belt acts as a member of the project team and reviews process improvements and the White Belt works in problem-solving teams as a beginner.

Six Sigma utilizes many qualitative and quantitative tools for process improvement, including statistical process control (SPC), control charts, process mapping, root cause analysis (RCA), and failure mode and effects analysis (FMEA). The main methodology Six Sigma uses is **DMAIC**, which stands for define, measure, analyze, improve, and control. This method lays out the steps for Six Sigma practitioners to follow, which begins with determining the problem and concludes by laying out long-term solutions. Although DMAIC is not the only methodology used by Six Sigma practitioners, it is by far one of the most common, and as such it is well-recognized. The target for quality performance in Six Sigma is only 3.4 defects or failures per million occurrences.

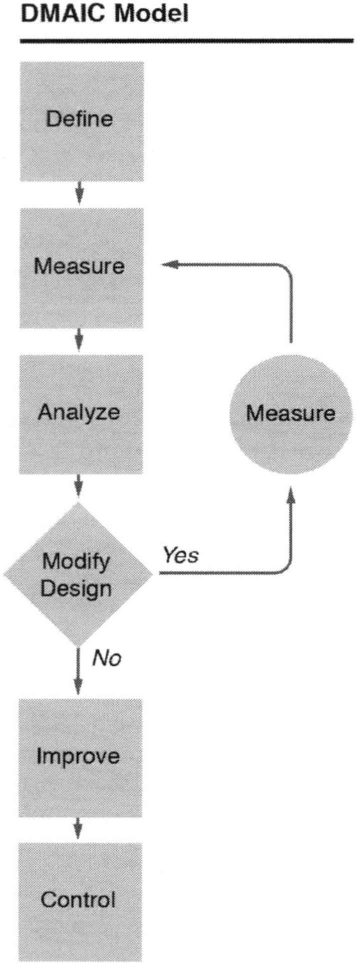


## Identifying Process Champions

Administrative leaders who are also team members may be referred to as **process champions**. These individuals should have the authority to grant the time and resources necessary to design and launch programs, as well as authority over areas that will be affected by the changes from those programs. Process champions are also responsible for coordinating internal communication with senior leadership, the Board of Directors, and staff members, and external communication with patients. The leadership provided by these process champions ensures that process improvement projects reach completion.

In addition to a process champion, a process improvement team may also have a primary care provider (PCP) champion. The PCP champion is a team member with a personal interest in improving a clinical process. This person may also assist in analyzing the program's metrics, to determine the success of different areas of the program, identify which areas are in need of improvement, and come up with solutions for those areas.

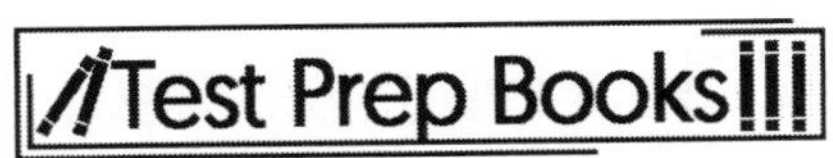

A process improvement champion should be proficient in business and operations, project selection, pacing, and results implementation. They should also have the following characteristics:

- Ability to envision and translate ideas into reality (strategic intelligence)
- Build culture by enacting values
- Alignment of business and social interests (social relevance)
- Instruct others in becoming leaders
- Create trust at all levels
- Developing mutually beneficial teamwork with external partners
- Distinguishing personal ideology and values from organizational practices and strategies

# *Implementation and Evaluation*

## Establishing Teams, Roles, Responsibilities, and Scope

It is often necessary to periodically evaluate processes to eliminate waste, remove redundancies, and reduce risks, while working to expand on the gains of currently successful practices. The implementation and evaluation processes include several key items. Key stakeholders and business leaders in healthcare organizations have an expectation of sustainable change, so the best approach is to be both innovative and imaginative. Once the parameters and goals of the project have been clearly defined, defects can be rooted out and eliminated. If the tactics are successful in their implementation, the end result will help to encourage agency-specific changes aligned with the mission, goals, and values of the host organization. The team seeks out opportunities to add value to the consumer experience and improve the overall experience.

In the rapidly-changing healthcare marketplace, intermittent evaluation of the effectiveness of an organization's culture is critical. Organizational excellence cannot be built if the departments, teams, and employees are not immersed in a culture that recognizes the importance of performance improvement standards. When the staff expects to be evaluated and rewarded for adherence to performance standards, the organization can become more competitive. It is also necessary for the leadership team to model being an effective team player. This top-down approach reinforces the company culture of competence and excellence. Moving from individual to collective accountability requires significant skill. Team-building efforts must result in a cohesive team. It is crucial to qualify and quantify the effectiveness of team members, in order to emphasize the importance of a team approach to improving current policies, procedures, and processes. When employees feel that their contribution is linked to the mission, values, and goals of the host organization, they are more likely to accept responsibility for their results.

It is necessary to confirm the depth and breadth of each team member's knowledge base. Since direct management staff are typically well aware of the individual skill sets of their employees, they are frequently notified when the CPHQ professional must build a reasonable candidate pool for projects. Once assembled, the candidates are dispatched to their respective teams and the real work of team building can begin.

One particularly effective team-building technique is **Bruce Tuckman's model**. This model for team building focuses on forming, storming, norming, performing and adjourning. Initially, the manager will begin **forming** the team. The primary goal in this phase is to encourage discussion among colleagues. Team members are chosen based on the areas of expertise necessary to achieve optimal results.

Together, the team members will create the framework of the performance improvement plan (PIP). Next, the manager will need to quiet and calm the **storms**, or the naturally-occurring conflicts between different team members' communication styles. The goal of this step is to explain the stages of the process and confirm that each team member is aware of their expected contribution.

Mutual trust in the team is built as each team member begins to recognize their separate and collective strengths. Norming is next. **Norming** is when team members come to recognize each other's strengths and resolve their differences. Members are encouraged to assume responsibility for their assigned roles. The manager acts as scaffolding, keeping the team members on task and fostering more collaboration. The next stage in Tuckman's model is defined as **performing**. During this phase, the manager can begin to take a less direct role and delegate activities to team members. Essentially, letting them do it by themselves builds each team member's confidence, competence, and skill set, which will cement individual accountability. **Adjourning** is when the project comes to a close and the team moves on, appreciating and reflecting on their growth as a team.

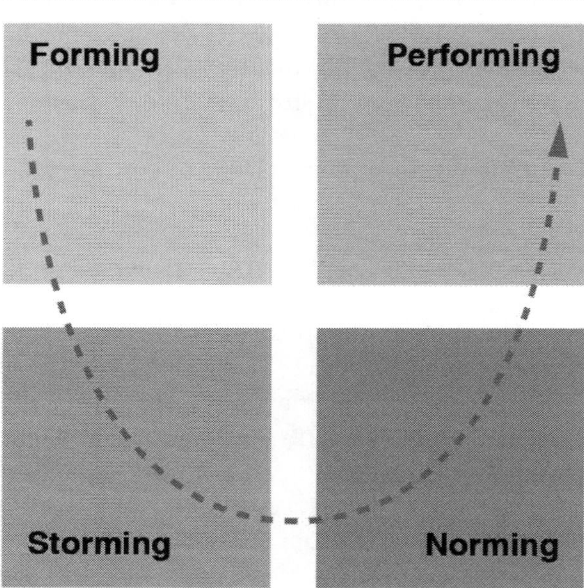


## Using a Range of Quality Tools and Techniques

When creating a blueprint for current policies and procedures, it is necessary to consider the most appropriate tools for the job. Depending on the scope of the project, the size of the organization, and the goals, the project management team must use certain tools to measure a baseline and terminal success. One of the most integral tools of an effective project management team is a commitment to cooperative and collaborative teamwork. Most project management teams use tools in the early phase of the project to define the limits of the intervention. Each rung of the process ladder is summarized or identified. The team creates the high-level process map, adding each individual facet of the processes as needed. The map reveals which steps need improvement. The process maps are typically designed as a

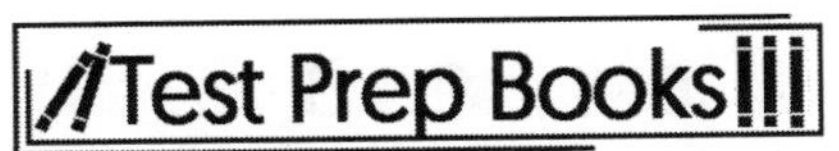

visual representation of the current processes, in an effort to find areas of redundancy and lack of value to the customer. This is always necessary to accomplish the goal of the project. Using clearly-labeled process maps, the team determines the basic definitions of the variables involved to accurately measure the problem.

An alternate form of program evaluation involves a more outcome-based method. Most CPHQ professionals work to determine how any given process in the system might fail. **Failure mode and effect analysis (FMEA)** seeks to uncover ways that business leaders can most effectively operationalize the efforts of frontline staff. The purpose is to find solutions before they become necessary. This form of program evaluation uses a qualitative approach to better understand and prevent future and ongoing threats to patient safety. The actual staff must be involved, as they can help to identify gaps in the practical application of the results. Both actual and perceived failures in practice are examined. Three questions are asked and answered:

- What is the severity of the effect on the customer?
- How often is this event likely to occur?
- How easily can the customer identify the problem?

Each category is ranked according to potential effect, severity of the effect, potential cause and probability of occurrence, and detection severity. Ranked in severity from 1 to 10 by the team, they are placed in descending order to begin the brainstorming portion of the problem-solving process. The assembled team will then begin working to create solutions to the identified problems. Wherever the actual failures are ranked as a 5 or greater, the risk assessment team will target how to implement the most effective solutions. The strategy continues with the team developing an action plan for erroneous or unnecessary steps in the current processes. As the momentum builds, more solutions become apparent.

One final format for depicting statistical data is the **fishbone**, or cause and effect diagram. Named precisely due to the shape, this diagram focuses largely on depicting the precipitating factors, or performing root cause analysis, for an event or outcome. Those root causes can then be separated into more meaningful categories. Practitioners can then periodically engage in the brainstorming and process mapping necessary to clarify potential solutions during each phase of the project. This format for evaluating the effectiveness of current processes is also useful in achieving results aligned with the objectives and value drivers of any organization.

## Project Timelines and Deliverables

Successful performance and process improvement requires the team to participate in monitoring of the timeline and deliverable objectives. As previously mentioned, the project team needs to determine the most necessary aspects of the initiative and align them with performance metrics. When performance metrics are reviewed, the focus can shift from problem-focused to solution-focused. The apparent gaps in outcomes related to the VOC and the VOB must be addressed and the staff retrained in an effort to standardize policies, procedures, and processes. The primary goal for process improvement in program evaluation is for the team to maintain the gains achieved by identifying statistically significant processes across the organization. The value added to the customer's experience is of paramount importance. This will encourage staff adherence to new process changes, thereby ensuring continued compliance and less variation. This continuation of the define stage of the DMAIC model encourages the team to ask a series of questions as listed below. The subsequent answers will be the driving force behind all the project charter initiatives.

- Which objectives must be accomplished first?
- What are the tangible deliverables for this project?
- What is the current state?
- What is the vision for the future state?
- How frequently will progress towards the goal be evaluated?
- How exactly will progress towards the ultimate goal be measured?
- What is the final due date for the project?
- What are the value-added benefits to the customer?

Simply put, performance and process improvement techniques focus on delivering value to the customer.

Performance and process improvement is essentially a game of remove and replace. Antiquated or ineffective processes are removed, and they are replaced with activities designed to increase the likelihood of success. The assembled project management team must define the projected outputs, or deliverables, to be received by the customer. Next, the team must determine whether the effort of the staff to implement the new processes is outweighed by the reward delivered to consumers. The cost-benefit analysis is an activity used in the Lean Six Sigma methodology as a way to determine the true costs of a potential solution compared to the actual benefits. It is frequently necessary to conduct a cost-benefit analysis at the start of the project charter, during the define phase, and throughout implementation of the project.

While working toward creating a cohesive plan of action, the key managers and decision-makers must be well aware of the KPIs. KPIs can best be defined as measurable data that will further indicate whether the goals are attainable. These performance measures enable the team to operationalize success. When considering what may go wrong, the team must determine whether the individual actions in the newly developed processes are logical. If the steps are too complex, they may be abandoned in favor of old habits. For this reason, mistake-proofing is used, which entails developing the necessary countermeasures to solve any problems before they actually occur. Although each activity in mistake-proofing can build on the previous step, the steps are also independent. Finally, the timeliness of the resolution of the PIP is crucial. Each initiative should have a measurable timeline, but performance improvement in the organization as a whole is an ongoing commitment to excellent performance. When performance improvement projects are considered as fluid in nature, it becomes evident that the periodic evaluation of their effectiveness is mandatory.

## Evaluating Team Effectiveness

It's important to keep track of team attendance. Late arrivals, early departures, and unusual patterns of sick days are all indicators that a team member's not meeting their maximum potential. There are several possible reasons for low attendance, including poor motivation, health issues, and burnout. These absences may put additional pressure on the rest of the team that has to pick up the slack for missing members. It's ideal to address issues of understaffing and overwork as early as possible to avoid risking the team's health and happiness.

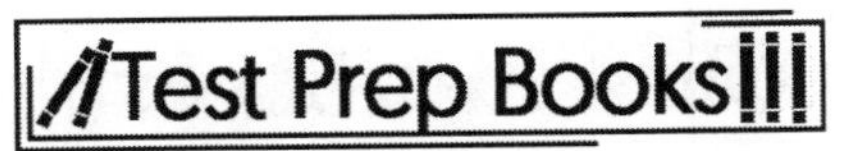

It's crucial that team members are able to finish their work on time. Ideally, they must be able to effectively prioritize tasks and have a thorough understanding of the time and resources available to them to complete their work efficiently. It's also important for organizations to identify team members that take initiative. Individuals who frequently take initiative are better suited for fast-paced workplaces that need employees to quickly adapt to changes and be proactive. Although it can be difficult to measure initiative-taking, the team leader may quantify how often a team member takes initiative. The most important, but most difficult, metric to define is the quality of a team member's work. Those who are invested in their work are more likely to achieve high levels of success, and it's important to recognize these achievements.

## Evaluating the Success of Performance Improvement Projects

A strong commitment to improving processes and employee performance improves the organization's ability to compete in the healthcare marketplace. Evaluating the success of performance improvement measures is integral to the maintenance of project management. Best practices of performance improvement include a willingness to seek a better understanding of the VOC, or voice of the patient, as well as the VOB. It is the critical examination of the answers to these questions that will guide the expansion of the process improvement implementation from general to specific goals and change the level of difficulty for measuring the effectiveness of the interventions from problematic to less challenging. It will always be more advantageous to consider the importance of adding to, rather than detracting from, the value delivered to customers.

Developed by Everett Rogers in 1962, the **theory of the Diffusion of Innovation** tries to explain how ideas and technology spread over time. Innovation is the action or process of developing a new idea, methodology, or action that improves on its predecessor. As it applies to performance improvement, diffusion can be defined as the passive and unplanned spread of new practices. This diffusion is said to occur through a **five-step decision-making process** containing the following steps: knowledge, persuasion, decision, implementation, and confirmation.

- **Knowledge**: When the individual is exposed to a new idea but lacks information about it.
- **Persuasion**: The individual is interested in the new idea and pursues information about it.
- **Decision**: The individual weighs the advantages/disadvantages and a decision is made about whether or not to accept the new idea.
- **Implementation**: The individual uses the new idea during this stage and determines its usefulness.
- **Confirmation**: The individual decides whether or not to continue using the new idea.

Effective performance improvement techniques involve training all groups in the organization. Managers must always remain diligent and remain aware that the responses of the process innovators, early adopters, and the early majority will most likely determine the success of the newly developed process and performance expectation. Once it has been determined which of the newly developed process modifications have been adopted, and to what degree, it will be necessary to determine their success.

The most necessary step in evaluating the success of process improvement is the execution of the pilot study. Participants in the pilot study need to be polled regarding their overall experience with the processes, the software, and any unexpected outcomes. It is crucial to engage with the members of the team, both individually and as a group. Which participants were responsible for encouraging other team members to endorse, adopt, and execute the process changes? Who are the process champions? How long did it take to integrate the changes in with current procedures? What, specifically, did the innovators perceive to be most effective? In what ways did the proposed process changes fail? During the improve phase of the DMAIC model, the goal is to assimilate all the ideas into a strategic plan that prioritizes opportunities for improvement. Additionally, the goal is to amend all processes associated with changes, including any process flows and job aids. Questions must be asked and answered in order for the team to adequately determine the most logical steps to document the agreed-upon process changes and improvements.

## Documenting Performance and Process Improvement Results

The ultimate goal for the team professional is to empower the organization's leadership to improve their employees' performance. Strategies that are no longer effective in bringing out the best in their employees must be replaced. Performance improvement planning also requires the team to collaborate with the leadership team and guide the development of a multidimensional approach that capitalizes on the internal strengths of the organization and minimizes weaknesses. During the control phase of the DMAIC model, the team needs to implement strategies to determine the sustainability and benefits of the newly defined processes. The team looks for feasible answers to the questions asked in the improve phase.

Monitoring and reviewing the process improvement project consists of assembling the team to review all the findings associated with the pilot study and the subsequent brainstorming sessions. Lessons learned through streamlining the ill-fitting portions of the new process will be applied. The project manager must periodically assess whether the team is on task, and it is also crucial to collect the lessons learned during each phase. This is most effective during the break-out brainstorming sessions, and once the managers have been trained on the newly developed processes.

The evaluation team will also return to review the issue logs and initiate thought process mapping, to further eliminate wasteful steps. How will gains be maintained? Have periodic process audits been established to assess the use and effectiveness of the solutions to ensure that staff do not revert to previous activities? In what ways have the results been leveraged to prevent occurrences of similar issues in all departments impacted by the problem? What is the most effective display of the findings? In an effort to prevent a recurrence of previously identified defects, the team must verify that the outcome of their action plan is functional, and they must further validate that the outcomes are aligned with the predetermined targets. Verification refers to testing that the proposed solution produces the desired outcome, while validation is a process that ensures that the outcome actually solves the problem. Once the results of the initial project are confirmed, a new project is identified, and the process begins again with the next identified issue of the organization.

The team must maintain an awareness of the nature of performance and process improvement. The goal is to train the leadership teams on the best practices to conduct performance and process improvement reviews periodically, utilizing the most effective methods. Once proficient in the Lean Six Sigma methodology, trained leaders become trainers themselves. The professional accountability and adherence to ongoing performance and process improvement measures afford the chosen organization the opportunity to remain competitive in the healthcare marketplace.

# Practice Quiz

1. Which of the following elements is NOT typically included in the project charter?
    a. Problem statement
    b. Process map
    c. Stakeholder analysis
    d. Goal statement

2. Which is *NOT* one of the five principles of lean thinking?
    a. Empowerment
    b. Flow and pull
    c. Employee satisfaction
    d. Perfection

3. During which stage of team development do team members find it relatively easy to be part of the team and can be seen taking on various roles and responsibilities as needed?
    a. Performing
    b. Forming
    c. Norming
    d. Adjourning

4. During which stage of team development might a team member be impolite when expressing frustrations about expectations toward another team member?
    a. Performing
    b. Storming
    c. Norming
    d. Forming

5. Which role assists the team when disputes arise in a project, encourages members to voice their opinions, and helps the parties involved move beyond an impasse by collaborating effectively?
    a. Project champion
    b. Process owner
    c. Facilitator
    d. Sponsor

**See answers on next page.**

# Answer Explanations

**1. B:** A process map typically isn't included in the project charter. Process maps are usually constructed later, as a tool within the project.

**2. C:** Employee satisfaction is *NOT* one of the five principles of lean thinking. The five principles include: value, creating a value stream, flow and pull, empowerment, and perfection.

**3. A:** During the performing stage of team development, team members find it relatively easy to be part of the team and can be seen taking on various roles and responsibilities as needed. During the forming stage, members have a great deal of uncertainty about the team's leadership, structure, and purpose. During the norming stage, the team members begin to grow closer to one another and respect the team leader as an authority figure. Finally, the adjourning stage involves wrapping up the team's activities.

**4. B:** During the storming stage of team development, a team member may be impolite when expressing frustrations about expectations toward another team member. During the performing stage of team development, team members find it relatively easy to be part of the team and can be seen taking on various roles and responsibilities as needed. During the norming stage, the team members begin to grow closer to one another and respect the team leader as an authority figure. Finally, during the forming stage, members have a great deal of uncertainty about the team's leadership, structure, and purpose.

**5. C:** A facilitator is the individual who assists the team when disputes arise in a Six Sigma project, encourages members to voice their opinions, and aides the parties involved to move beyond an impasse by collaborating effectively. The project champion essentially owns the project. They are charged with ensuring the project's success and representing the organization's interests. This individual is involved in the activities of project selection, project kickoff (in conjunction with the project leader), and providing overall support to and communicating with the project team. The process owner is the individual who's responsible for the business process which is the focus of the Six Sigma project. Finally, the sponsor is the senior executive who's supporting the Six Sigma movement within the company.

# Patient Safety

## *Assessment and Planning*

### Assessing the Organization's Culture of Safety

Effective program evaluation begins with an in-depth assessment of all aspects associated with the safety of the organization. The role of a healthcare quality professional is the evaluation and ongoing review of the quality of patient safety within healthcare settings. A focus on safety is not merely the avoidance of errors. Patient safety has to be considered in every aspect of care. The healthcare quality professional confirms which policies and procedures are practical, which are outdated or ineffective, and which need to be revised.

The primary goal of patient safety is the prevention of harm through the methodical analysis of previously harmful events. This is accomplished through the systematic review of those policies and procedures both directly and indirectly related to patient safety. For example, when evaluating the provision of bedside care in a hospital setting, it is essential to assess the official and unofficial procedures of the nursing staff. This can be accomplished through shadowing randomly selected nurses and healthcare providers on multiple shifts, medical record reviews, and incident reports. Is the patient handoff conducted at the bedside, or does it frequently occur at the nurse's station? Do nurses scan the patient's wristband with each scheduled administration of medications? It is also important to ensure this culture of safety is apparent not only to clinical staff, but also to ancillary providers and the patients themselves.

Initially, the healthcare quality professional examines the organization's core mission and values. One of the most influential aspects of promoting a culture of patient safety is to assess the attitude exhibited by organizational leadership. It is the leadership team that will ultimately develop the core culture. The primary goal of this portion of the assessment is to determine if the organizational culture is an accurate reflection of the initial vision of the organization. How clearly are the core values articulated to the staff? Do the policies and procedures reflect the proposed core mission and values? How does the leadership team respond to incidents that contradict the organization's core mission and values? What actions have been taken to perform periodic internal evaluations of the staff? Healthcare quality analysists must ascertain if an actual culture of safety exists within the organization and how visible it is to patients and staff. The next step is to ensure that the culture is reinforced and find ways to enhance it.

Policies and procedures enacted by healthcare organizations to ensure patient safety typically include factors that meet The Joint Commission National Patient Safety goals. The Joint Commission established the **National Patient Safety (NPS)** goals in 2002 and implemented them the following year. This nationwide effort instituted a set of uniform, realistic, and specific goals that could be consistently applied and measured in every healthcare setting. National Patient Safety goals have set the standard for excellence and are set annually. Several of the most important goals applicable in every healthcare setting include: identifying patients correctly, using medications safely, preventing infection, identifying patient safety risks, and improving staff communications.

Each goal requires that the leadership create an atmosphere of patient-centered care, with a focus on the interdepartmental teamwork necessary to maintain the safety of the entire patient population. Any breech in patient security should be noted, along with recommendations on the necessary adjustments. Accreditation assumes that every healthcare agency seeking recognition is interested in developing the types of programs, policies, and procedures that focus on evidence-based, clinically appropriate care. Physicians, nurses, and other healthcare providers view the accreditation of an institution as a sign of excellence. Other benefits can include the fact that many local and state governments reward healthcare organizations for being recognized through expedited licensure, waivers through Medicare and Medicaid, third-party reimbursement, and improved access to more lucrative managed care contracts.

## Determining How Technology Can Enhance the Patient Safety Program

Medical records were not kept and maintained until the early 1920s, when physicians realized the importance of a patient's medical history when providing care. This practice was helpful, but patient histories were often incomplete and rarely accessible by other healthcare providers. Simply storing the numerous documents required entire rooms and often whole floors of hospitals and offices. It wasn't until the late 1960s when the first computer was created that the healthcare sector began to consider the widespread use of computers. Since the earliest computers were cumbersome and expensive, their use was common only in large hospitals and government agencies. The 1970s ushered in a need for more extensive medical record keeping. With the influx of American veterans returning home and needing significant medical and psychiatric care, paper medical files were largely traded in for computerized records. The introduction of President Obama's American Recovery and Reinvestment Act of 2009 required at least 70% of all healthcare organizations transition to electronic medical records by 2014.

The **electronic health record**, or **EHR**, is one of the primary tools utilized in the maintenance of patient safety. Within many healthcare settings, the EHR is easily accessible to physicians, pharmacists, nurses, and other ancillary providers. This allows for each individual involved in caring for a specific patient to be immediately aware of any changes in diagnoses, medications, allergies, and treatments. Medications entered hastily are flagged when contradictory information, such as other medications or allergies, is noted by the sophisticated medical software. The majority of larger medical facilities have further incorporated bedside charting for all providers so that information can be easily updated in the patient's room, and wristbands are scanned prior to medication administration to confirm that appropriate medications are dispensed.

One pitfall of the electronic medical record involves the human factor. Since a computer is only capable of providing information based on what is entered, information entered inaccurately or omitted has the potential to harm a patient. Consider a patient who enters an emergency room with an acute allergic reaction to a new medication. If the hospital is not a part of the healthcare system that the patient typically frequents, this information may not be readily available in the electronic record. This opens the door for inaccurate patient records and the possibility of harm to the patient. For these reasons, numerous companies have software specifically developed to safeguard electronic medical records. Currently, those safeguards often include extensive firewalls, applications that require rolling and random password changes, multiple tiers of medical record access, and closed network connections.

Additional technological security measures that have been instituted in healthcare organizations include those created for infants and patients managing mental health concerns. The majority of labor and delivery, nursery, and mother-baby units within hospitals are equipped with technologically enhanced abduction protocols. When admitted to the labor and delivery unit, expectant mothers receive a regular

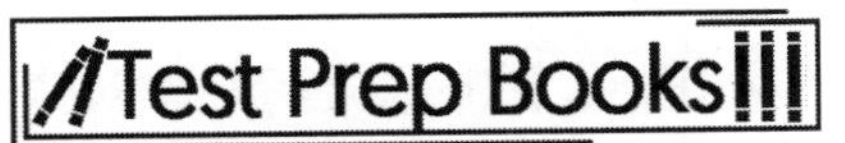

hospital wristband with a patient identification number. Once the infant is born, they also receive a similar ankle bracelet with the corresponding mother's name and their own patient identification number; this number is also connected with the medical records of the birth mother.

Infants must travel in a bassinette and are always accompanied by medical personnel from their respective units in the hospital. Once reunited with the birth mother, both arm bands are scanned, to confirm that both the mother and child are related through the patient identification numbers. The ankle bracelet is also equipped with an alarm that will sound and disable all points of egress from the unit, to prevent abduction. A similar alert wristband is used for inpatient mental health units, those admitted from correctional facilities, or those at risk for suicide. Patients at risk for elopement are prevented from exiting the floor or entering elevators. Other rooms are equipped with cameras that continually monitor patients. Overall, the technological improvements and changes are necessary to guard the protected health information of all patients.

## Participating in Risk Management Assessment Activities

It is essential to maintain strict guidelines regarding quality and patient safety. Patient safety specialists often need to collaborate with the risk management team, quality department, patient advocates, infection prevention, and members of the board of ethics. Quality professionals must have an intimate knowledge of healthcare organizations and accreditation standards, and they must possess the ability to apply them. **The Joint Commission of Healthcare Organizations** was officially formed in 1951 as a formalized and structured way to monitor patient safety in healthcare settings. Currently, The Joint Commission accredits, or recognizes, over 20,000 hospitals, nursing homes, and other healthcare organizations on the quality of care that they provide. The overall mission of this nonprofit association is to independently examine the policies and procedures that threaten patient safety, and it has become the gold standard of evidence-based medical care.

Risk management professionals employ multiple tactics to evaluate patient safety in healthcare organizations. The three main principles of risk management assessment are risk assessment, risk avoidance, and risk control. **Risk assessment** is the initial and most important step in the process. What happened and why? The analyst will need access to all available records, participants, policies, and procedures associated with the event. Methodical and purposeful deconstruction of every step should be mapped, and any discrepancies in processes, hardware, human factors, and organizational culture scrutinized. Similar incidents and associated resolutions within other healthcare settings should be compared and analyzed for probability of success. The avoidance of future risk forms the foundation for the next step: the analyst's review of the plan for potential vulnerabilities. What specific actions, policies, and procedures would prevent this type of incident in the future? What safeguards need to be in place at various stages in related procedures to undergird current processes? Finally, the risk management team develops measures to increase quality of care through the adaptation of specific control measures. The following example highlights the application of this strategy:

A patient admitted for a below-the-knee amputation of the left leg reported a concern to the nursing manager. According to the patient, the physician entered the room, discussed the procedure, and marked the right leg for the procedure. When the patient protested, the physician advised him that the medical chart indicated the right leg as the limb to be removed. When the patient continued to protest and refused to sign the consent form for the incorrect limb, the physician cancelled the surgery and left the room angrily. When the nursing manager reviewed additional patient records, it was revealed that the patient had been correct; somehow, the medical record had been updated incorrectly the previous evening. The patient had developed a decubitus ulceration on the right heel, which was scheduled for debridement. The physician that reviewed the notes assumed that the right limb, not the left, would be removed. The nurse manager consulted the physician, and the surgery was rescheduled for the correct limb. A risk management team was assembled to review this near-miss event and it became clear that there was a miscommunication during the patient handoff from the surgical resident to the attending surgeon.

Two issues were noted during the risk assessment: The policy to conduct patient report at the bedside was not followed, and the correct limb was not marked per NPS guidelines. This incident could be avoided in the future by following established procedures regarding surgery time out. To control the likelihood of this event being repeated, the quality professional proposed that the surgical team receive additional training regarding the time-out requirements and procedures regarding bedside report. Continued education credits were provided to clinical staff as part of their annual continuing education requirements. Finally, the leadership team released a facility-wide newsletter, which included a brief synopsis of the event and the NPS guidelines regarding bedside report and surgery time out. The next step is to facilitate ongoing adherence to new patient safety guidelines.

# *Implementation and Evaluation*

## Facilitating the Ongoing Evaluation of Safety Activities

One of the most significant and effective practices that healthcare quality professionals can employ in risk assessment is the Lean Six Sigma method. Although initially developed in the manufacturing sector, the Lean Six Sigma method of assessing and managing risk has taken root in healthcare. Any deviation from the standard processes typically results in higher risks to the patient. The basic principles of Lean Six Sigma in relation to the management of decreasing risks to patient safety include:

- Define the expected outcome
- Measure the actual versus perceived risk
- Analyze the scope of the risk to patients
- Improve the typical versus the most-desirable outcomes
- Control the ongoing risks to patients

When improvement is required for existing processes, Lean Six Sigma helps to define, measure, analyze, improve, and control quality—or DMAIC—with staff empowered to collect the data. The **DMAIC model** allows for the methodical development of an action plan to streamline and standardize laborious processes, reduce waste, and mitigate risks to the patient population in any healthcare setting. One additional outflow in this process is to consider the Lean 5S method: sort, simplify, sweep, standardize, self-discipline. The priority for this facet of Lean Six Sigma is to teach the leadership team the importance of improving simplification. This exercise encourages managers and executives to model ways to remove all nonessential items in their work environment. The exercise informs their understanding of the adjustments required of front-line staff. All are emboldened to offer strategies that remove redundant processes, while increasing focus on what is vital.

In the initial step, Lean Six Sigma professionals partner with the leadership of healthcare organizations and their risk management team to create an assessment of current processes. The team then works to create a process map, formulate problem and goal statements, and identify the specific needs of patients and medical staff. This approach is solution focused, and unidirectional. Each interdepartmental

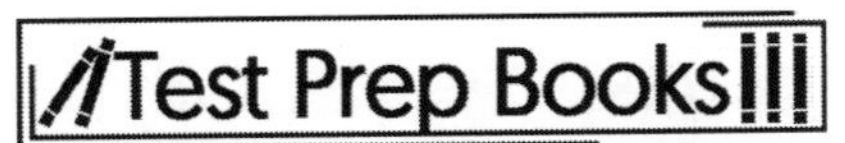

connection is assessed for interruptions in current processes. Raw quantitative data, in the form of near-miss and sentinel events, are gathered and analyzed. Incident reports are also reviewed in an effort to backtrack and pinpoint any breakdowns in processes, areas for improving the skillset of each employee, and ways to increase the quality of care provided. Process maps are compared with actual staff activities and then restructured around the new, more practical solutions. Finally, the team will work with leadership to ensure that the new response plan is effective and discuss methods to integrate new processes throughout the organization.

## Integrating Safety Concepts Throughout the Organization

Upon completion of the analysis of any near-miss or sentinel event, the findings must be integrated into the current policies and procedures. Controlling the incidence and prevalence of sentinel events involves implementing practices that also improve the quality of care provided to patients. Technological advances in medical care have dramatically impacted healthcare delivery and overall patient safety. From the EHR to abduction and elopement security systems to smart medication pumps, innovations can either enhance or endanger overall patient safety. Proponents of patient safety often speak to the benefits of utilizing technology to augment current processes. Accurate record keeping allows quality specialists to protect the interests of the organization and the patient. Tracking the incidence and prevalence of near-miss and sentinel events is vital to meeting local and governmental regulations. The leadership team is responsible for organizing, coordinating, and facilitating the development of programs that control the clinical risks associated with patient care services in healthcare organizations. The organization must periodically conduct utilization reviews to uncover documentation irregularities. Most often, safety audits begin with reviews of patient medical records; this necessitates the importance of the standardization of documentation in the legal medical records.

Patient safety has become synonymous with risk management. Unfortunately, despite the numerous safeguards, individuals evaluating the level of care that patients receive must develop practices that confront those risks. Quality control specialists require extensive knowledge in the management of patient relations and how to de-escalate conflict. Communication skills, team building, and leadership effectiveness are all integral to the maintenance of established patient safety goals.

Risk management agents work diligently to ensure that the medical treatments patients receive do not result in associated risks. They are trained to evaluate the potential for harm as well as the causes for real events. They act when near-miss or sentinel events occur and periodically review national statistics in an effort to prevent future incidents. Whenever a healthcare provider engages in activities that contradict the current policies and procedures of the organization, those actions can and often do result in actual or potential harm to the patient. Emphasis remains on how to design and alter work processes to focus on safety, quality, and improved performance standards for the hospital system. The ultimate goal of the integration of risk management and quality control in healthcare program evaluation is to streamline current processes in favor of more efficient and effective methods.

## Using Safety Principles

Professionals that examine the principles of patient safety and quality management use qualitative and quantitative data to measure the impact of errors in healthcare delivery. **Qualitative research** in risk management yields data in the form of concepts, which gives insight and understanding to contributing factors. **Quantitative investigation** reveals raw numbers, which are then typically translated into more familiar and relatable terms. The EHR forced facilities to install costly software with no guarantee that it would meet their needs. Numerous firewalls and passwords cannot always prevent basic human error when data are entered. High-reliability organizations often flourish in adversity with above-average security measures. Proponents of systems analysis combine the deeper dive with a broad view and tie all of the factors together. Critical analysis of each element within the system facilitates improved functioning of the organization as a whole. Each form of data is combined to further the goal of increasing patient safety.

It is important to consider the ethical and financial cost of breaches in patient safety. Adverse events within healthcare organizations results in a loss of credibility for a particular organization, but also can be catastrophic to the entire healthcare industry. Hospitals may lose the confidence of patients and may even face excessive financial losses. Failures to address the root cause and the subsequent effects of near-miss and sentinel events profoundly affect the patients and medical staff, extended families, friends, and society. The more significant the event is, the higher the likelihood of the offending organization dissolving.

Using an ongoing team approach develops strategies for predicting and preventing the incidence of sentinel and near-miss events. Evidence-based practice has revealed that certain principles, when followed, improve overall patient safety. Although no specific method is significantly more valuable than any other; each has its own merit. The similarities of each technique can be found in the shared goals of enhancing the overall culture of safety, and the mitigation of risk to patients. Techniques such as systems thinking and introducing the methods associated with high-reliability organizations have produced significant advances in risk management.

## Human-Factors Engineering

**Human-factors engineering**, also known as **ergonomics**, is a discipline that develops devices and technology based on the physical and psychological needs of those who use them. This field combines technological advances in healthcare with the specific needs of humans in mind.

As an example, the nurse manager of a thirty-bed medical surgical unit was advised of a near-miss medication error for an elderly patient receiving hypertensive medications. Although the error was caught before the patient received the medication, the director of nursing assembled a risk management team to review the case. The patient had been admitted earlier that morning, was transferred to the inpatient unit after an episode of syncope at a local skilled nursing facility, and the attending physician requested that the patient be admitted for a head computed tomography (CT) scan to determine if any head injury had occurred. The patient's diagnoses included Alzheimer's disease and hypertension. The patient was nonverbal, and no family members were available at the time of the admission. The patient was admitted with the same medication list, but the attending physician called in additional orders at the time of admission. Orders to discontinue the hypertensive medications to rule out hypotension as a cause for the fall were not transcribed or discussed during the transition of care to the next nurse. This example underscores the human factors involved in evaluating patient safety activities. Human fallibility is the cause for this near miss.

Human-factors engineering focuses on how to build technology through usability testing, forcing functions, and as a work around. Usability explains how the device is used in a real-world situation. Forcing functions prevents one step from being completed without a prior necessary step. This case presents an opportunity to enhance patient handoffs, encourage immediate order transcription, or to institute a policy adding a secondary nurse to electronically cosign medication administration at the

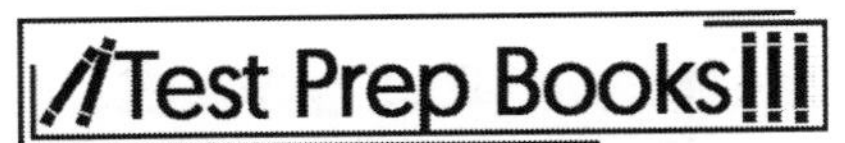

bedside. This event also presents an opportunity for departmental leadership to offer training and discussion regarding the importance of highlighting the overall culture of quality within the department.

## High Reliability

There are five specific factors that make operating as a high-reliability organization advantageous: reliance on practical experience, loyalty in adversity, an outcome-focused approach, an emphasis on operationalized definitions of expected outcomes, and a deeper-dive perspective when unexpected problems arise. Organizations that adopt this method of risk management achieve a high level of excellence because they focus on anticipating the best response to the worst-case scenario.

The Joint Commission has established benchmarks for quality that drive the high-reliability organization to consistently anticipate probable threats to patient safety. This model also provides transparency, accountability, and shared responsibility within the organization that reinforces problem solving. It also increases facility-wide awareness of new initiatives that reinforce patient safety. Equipped with this qualitative approach to risk management, the leadership team can prepare to follow the data points where they lead. These occurrences are not desired, but they are used as opportunities.

A sentinel event involving the death of a patient in an intensive care unit, after an anaphylactic reaction to a hastily administered blood transfusion, can be examined using the standard high-reliability approach. Facilities that utilize this approach would begin with a roundtable discussion to reveal the basic facts of the incident. Critical care nurses who routinely infuse blood, as well as emergency room nurses, would serve as the practical experts in this case. The nurse in question would not be abandoned but educated on the best practices as evidenced by the techniques of more experienced colleagues. Their collective experience can help shed light on which procedural steps were missed or how current practices may be inadequate. A more in-depth exploration of the contributing factors, and a focus on established procedures, helps to expose gaps in current processes. Once uncovered, the risk management team can begin to work quickly to find the solution.

## Systems Thinking

**Systems thinking** involves a more holistic approach to risk management assessment. One main goal is to understand how the different parts of the whole system work together. While typical program evaluation tends to compartmentalize, this approach investigates each incident based on how the separate systems within the hospital network have influenced an outcome. This method deconstructs the incident without an expected conclusion. Systems thinking involves asking two questions. How does each separate system contribute to the problem? In what ways can each system contribute to the solution? Recognizing that each department is itself a subsystem, equally dependent on the other departments, exposes the complex relationship as it relates to the whole. It is impossible to provide excellent care to patients without the interdependency of the entire facility.

Systems thinking also enlists cognitive mapping as a way to represent physical locations. Areas where each subsystem perceives its connections to the others can help identify still more points of interaction that contributed to the sentinel event. Does each separate department have the capacity to identify and accept responsibility for their contribution to the problem? Quality experts are also assembled for the purpose of integrating departmental perspectives to identify patterns. Often, these unexpected results help to formulate a cohesive picture of how the system has broken down.

Systems thinking is also vital in building confidence throughout the organization. The ability to rely on each individual department to demand individual and collective responsibility for their own parts in the process sets the stage for interdepartmental transparency and accountability. Systems thinking challenges antiquated and inadequate processes to protect the patient population of any healthcare setting.

## Participating in Safety and Risk Management Activities

### Incident Report Review

The first step is to read the incident report. After that, the nurses and other staff involved must be interviewed. Did the nurse follow every step in the established protocol? Is it possible that the nurse may have been overtired or overextended with too many patients? Staffing models should be examined to determine if the nurse-to-patient ratios are adequate for each shift. In this instance, clinical quality specialists must collaborate with clinical and administrative personnel to create a workable plan of action. Once the required information has been gathered, the next step is to present the findings for the leadership of the organization to conduct a final review and root-cause analysis.

### Sentinel/Unexpected Event Review

A **sentinel event** is an unforeseen occurrence that results in actual harm or death to a patient or a group of patients. In Healthcare risk management, an action or inaction that may have resulted in nonlethal injury to a patient is known as a near-miss event. Once uncovered, a near-miss or sentinel incident highlights the policies and procedures that resulted in the error. Risk management assessments must also involve an examination of problematic behaviors within the organization that foster an unsafe environment. Simply updating obsolete policies or procedures cannot completely mitigate risk. It is often necessary to deconstruct hierarchies, review organizational management charts, leadership attitudes, and the overall culture of safety. **Adverse events** are often associated with debilitating injuries, and the risk management team can employ various techniques to analyze the actual and potential causes of the events. Formal and informal nursing practices are scrutinized, as habitual behaviors can lead to complacency. Quality and patient safety professionals then evaluate the current departmental and accreditation standards. Once it is determined which areas do not meet or exceed evidence-based standards and practices, a full risk management team is assembled to establish more effective protocols.

The risk management team must consist of individuals who value the organizational structure as much as they value patient safety. Medical records, incident reports, and at least one completely objective healthcare quality professional must be involved. The review panel must also include a representative from the internal ethical review board. This will ensure an accurate appraisal of the ethical implications of the incident. It will be necessary to determine which steps in the protocol led to the near-miss or sentinel event, and at which point the risk assessment team could intervene in order to prevent a recurrence of a similar incident.

### Root-Cause Analysis

**Root-cause analysis** is used to evaluate patient safety in healthcare organizations. The tool identifies the underlying causes of sentinel and near-miss events and helps develop safeguards to prevent the recurrence of the incidents. In a root-cause analysis, a healthcare quality evaluator asks a series of "why" questions regarding the incident. This process is implemented to sift through current policies and reveal causal factors within the control of the team. Patient factors are not included in this step. The team must be able to influence the root cause for the modifications to be successful. The analyst must determine a causal factor from a root cause. Although some events are identified through the detection

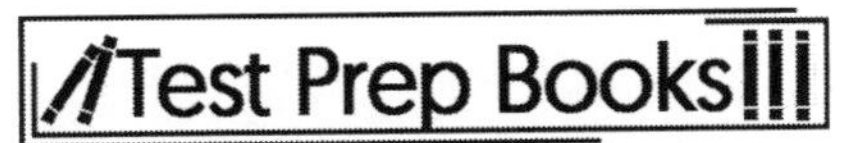

of a near miss, a sentinel event, or an incident report, other causes may involve employees or patients requesting a resolution. This systemic approach does not insist solely upon individual accountability, but rather a consideration of areas of improvement within the organization.

Consider the following example regarding the analysis of a near-miss event, and how this event can be avoided in future interactions:

A patient being treated in an urgent care clinic was almost given a medication that would have caused an anaphylactic allergic reaction. Utilizing the "five why's," it was determined that there were multiple contributing factors. Several nurses were out sick with the flu, causing higher nurse-to-patient ratios; the nurse involved had a total of ten patients, which is more than double the allowable ratio of one-to-four ratio for the clinic. Although the nurse had received the appropriate orders from the attending physician regarding the medications, it was a verbal order, which the overextended nurse failed to transcribe. This led to a failure to add the new medication to the electronic medical record. The failure to adhere to the safeguard of scanning wristbands to retrieve the computerized medication was a significant breech in the quality of care. Interdepartmental breakdowns in staffing models, protocols for vaccinations of nursing staff (which does not replace viral control), and policies for accepting verbal orders could have all influenced this near miss. This root-cause analysis opens the dialogue to examine the best methods to verify improvement once the new processes are implemented.

## Failure Mode and Effects Analysis

An alternate form of program evaluation involves a more outcome-based method. Quality and safety professionals work to determine how any given process within the system might fail. **Failure mode and effect analysis** is not a quantitative approach but does seek to uncover ways the departments can operationalize their efforts. The purpose is to find solutions before they are needed. This form of program evaluation enlists a qualitative approach to better understand and prevent future and ongoing threats to patient safety. The actual staff must be involved, as they can help identify gaps in the practical application of the results. Both actual and perceived failures in practice are examined. Three specific questions are asked and answered:

- What is the severity of the effect on the patient?
- How often is this event likely to occur?
- How easily can the patient independently identify the problem?

Each category is ranked by potential effect, severity of the effect, the potential cause and probability of occurrence, and detection severity. Ranked in severity from 1 to 10 by the team, they are placed in descending order to begin the brainstorming portion of the problem-solving process. The assembled team then begins working to create solutions to the identified problems. Wherever the actual failures rank as a 5 or greater, the risk assessment team targets how to implement the most effective solutions. The process continues with the team developing an action plan and as momentum builds, more solutions become apparent. Quality analysts then examine the evidence within the incident report and compare the findings to similar events. Gaps in processes are filled and strengths leveraged within the system to prevent future recurrence of the event. The success of the intervention is determined by process improvement and evidenced by a lower incidence of comparable events.

# Practice Quiz

1. Which of the following is the best way to prevent the spread of infection?
    a. Keeping the mouth covered when coughing or sneezing
    b. Disinfecting shared patient equipment
    c. Practicing proper hand hygiene
    d. Avoiding contact with infectious patients

2. Which of the following is now considered synonymous with risk management?
    a. Sentinel events
    b. Systems thinking
    c. Ergonomics
    d. Patient safety

3. Which of the following tools would NOT be used to determine why goals were not achieved or why there was a discrepancy between expected outcomes and actual outcomes?
    a. Six Sigma
    b. Gap analysis
    c. Root cause analysis
    d. Cause-and-effect diagram

4. Processes should be audited regularly to ensure they are providing the same results and outcomes consistently. What method monitors a process from start to finish to ensure the same results occur every time?
    a. Transparency
    b. Validation
    c. Data collection
    d. Risk management

5. During a Failure Mode and Effects Analysis (FMEA), each category is ranked by all EXCEPT which of the following?
    a. The potential cause and probability of occurrence
    b. The cost of rectifying the cause
    c. The severity of the effect
    d. The potential effect

**See answers on next page.**

# Answer Explanations

**1. C:** All of the answer choices are types of standard precautions, but research has shown that proper hand hygiene using soap and water or alcohol-based hand rub (if appropriate) is the best way to prevent the spread of germs.

**2. D:** Patient safety has become synonymous with risk management. Prioritizing patient safety in all cases is critical in preventing injuries.

**3. A:** Six Sigma is a specific technique that works to improve business processes by implementing various tools and concepts to reduce errors and eliminate waste. Gap analysis, root cause analysis, and cause-and-effect diagrams, Choices *B, C,* and *D,* are incorrect because they are all tools that would be used to determine why goals were not achieved or if there was a discrepancy between the expected results and actual results.

**4. B:** Validation is the auditing method used to ensure that a process delivers the same outcomes each time it is used. Validation looks at each step within a process to ensure consistency and predictability. Choice *A,* transparency, is a vital component of communication that builds trust. Choice *C,* data collection, refers to the specific process of sourcing information. Choice *D,* risk management, is the process that identifies potential risks within a process.

**5. B:** When conducting a FMEA, each category is ranked by potential effect, severity of the effect, the potential cause and probability of occurrence, and detection severity. The cost of fixing the potential issue is not considered. Ranked in severity from 1 to 10 by the team, the categories are placed in descending order to begin the brainstorming portion of the problem-solving process.

# Practice Test #1

1. When preliminary denial of accreditation by TJC requires the organization to provide additional detail, when must the organization provide the information?
   a. Within one month
   b. Within ten working days
   c. Before the end of the current survey
   d. Before the end of the current month

2. Which statement best describes the Lean Six Sigma approach to process improvement?
   a. The Lean Six Sigma approach can be defined as the continual and collaborative discipline of measuring and comparing the results of key work processes
   b. A plan to eliminate or lower the likelihood of an error, or to make the occurrence of an error so obvious that any possibility of that error impacting the consumer is practically impossible
   c. The primary goal is to produce more effective processes, policies, and procedures that reduce variation and significantly lower the chances of negative outcomes
   d. A specific methodology that calculates the true costs of a potential solution compared to the actual benefits

3. What is the best definition for critical to quality measures (CTQs)?
   a. The correlation, or dependent relationship, between two quantitative continuous variables, whether positive or negative
   b. The necessary countermeasures to solve any problems before they actually occur
   c. The measurable data that will further indicate whether the goals and objectives are attainable
   d. The aspects of a business process or product that must be met in order to satisfy the consumer

4. What is the basis for The Joint Commission's adoption of the National Patient Safety Goals?
   a. To force healthcare organizations to prevent mistakes during surgical procedures
   b. To institute inflexible patient-safety measures to provide high-quality care
   c. To encourage healthcare organizations to institute high quality standards for patient safety
   d. To capitalize on the fees paid to The Joint Commission or accreditation

5. What is the most necessary step in evaluating the success of process improvement?
   a. Teamwork
   b. Executing the pilot study
   c. Informing administration of the plans
   d. An action plan

6. Which statement best describes the purpose of the project charter?
   a. The primary goal is to determine the ability of a specific process to deliver value as required by the customer.
   b. This written agreement usually includes the primary reason for the project, the goal and scope of the project, the expected budget, and the roles of each team member.
   c. The written agreement that acts as measurable data to indicate if the goals and objectives of the project are attainable.
   d. The primary goal is to produce more effective processes, policies, and procedures that reduce variation and significantly lower the chances of negative outcomes.

7. During strategic planning, what is the main task of the leadership team?
   a. To lead teams
   b. To act as clinical advisors
   c. To develop strategies
   d. To maintain records

8. Before sending out a meeting invite, what is the most important thing the facilitator must do?
   a. Decide who to have on the team
   b. Get approval from administration
   c. Define the objective of the meeting
   d. Set goals

9. Which is the best description for the acronym SIPOC?
   a. Supplier, inputs, process, outputs, customer
   b. Supporter, inputs, process, outcomes, consumer
   c. Supplier, improvement, product, outputs, consumer
   d. Supporters, inputs, products, outcomes, consumer

10. How does a healthcare risk management assessment typically begin?
   a. Interviewing the patient to get their reaction.
   b. Meeting with attorneys to discuss possible causes of the incident.
   c. Reviewing the incident report.
   d. Interviewing the leadership of the organization.

11. What is meant by fiduciary duty to care?
   a. Assurance that the board members of a healthcare organization are prudent, acting in good faith, and making decisions in the best interest of the organization
   b. A measure of the fiscal responsibility of the stakeholders within any healthcare organization
   c. Assurance that the board members of a healthcare organization are applying the specific, measurable, accurate, reliable, and timely (SMART) method of goal setting for the organization
   d. A measure of the ability of the CPHQ professional to control the costs of obtaining and maintaining accreditation and/or certification

12. What is the major advantage of using scorecards and dashboards during a process and performance improvement?
   a. Both are designed as a visual representation of the current processes, in an effort to find areas of redundancy and lacking in value to the customer.
   b. Using scorecards and dashboards during a performance review can help highlight areas where additional training around related processes and procedures is needed.
   c. The election and introduction of team members based on the areas of expertise helps to achieve optimal results.
   d. Both individual and collective contributions of employees are recognized, reinforcing the establishment of the newly developed skills.

13. How are credentialing and privileging different?
    a. Credentialing involves the oversight of licensing to medical professionals under their scope of practice; privileging refers to the evaluation of a practitioner's actual performance and qualifications.
    b. Credentialing is typically based on payment for the number of individuals a physician provides care for, whereas privileging is typically based on the quality of care provided.
    c. Privileging involves the oversight of licensing to medical professionals under their scope of practice; credentialing refers to the evaluation of a practitioner's actual performance and qualifications.
    d. Credentialing is the passive and unplanned span of new practices; privileging is the rate at which the new practices are adopted and implemented.

14. What is the major difference between scorecards and dashboards?
    a. Scorecards involve comparing equivalent processes within the same organization; dashboards can be comparing similar processes to a competitor within the same industry
    b. Scorecards are a single payment made to cover the costs of the treatment provided for any given treatment; dashboards are written agreements that act as measurable data to indicate if the goals and objectives of the project are attainable
    c. Scorecards can be defined as a written account that compares and measures the performance of specific individuals against the projected goals of the organization; dashboards are quality measurement tools that actually allow the management team to compare and contrast different reports or access diverse datasets in one place
    d. Scorecards can be defined as the passive and unplanned spread of new practices; dashboards are defined as the active spread of those new practices to a target audience utilizing planned methodologies

15. What is work performance data?
    a. A written document designed to be a visual roadmap for process improvement
    b. Measurable data that indicates whether the goals and objectives are attainable
    c. Raw data related to the occurrence of specific tasks.
    d. The dependent relationship between two quantitative continuous variables, either positive or negative.

16. Which of the following is true regarding data management?
    a. It is only done by IT personnel with education in data management
    b. It is always done on local servers within a hospital
    c. It is done via cloud based systems in a healthcare environment
    d. It involves acquiring, validating, storing, protecting, and processing data

17. Why should processes be evaluated frequently?
    a. To eliminate waste and reduce risk
    b. Because it is mandated by The Joint Commission
    c. To reinforce employee trainings
    d. To determine if they still work

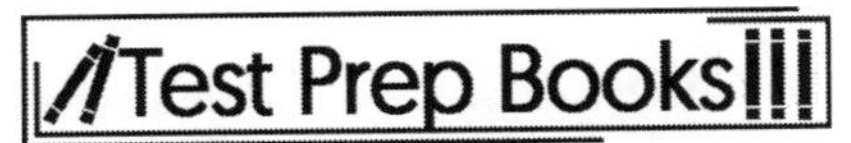

18. What is the leadership team's first action when preparing for a survey by an accreditation agency?
    a. To assemble all of the policy and procedure books
    b. To inform all the staff of the impending survey by email
    c. To engage staff in discussions regarding how each department has succeeded
    d. To begin writing an action plan

19. Which of the following statements is true regarding the policies and procedures for healthcare settings?
    a. They ensure patient safety and typically include factors that meet The Joint Commission National Patient Safety goals.
    b. Many focus on developing devices and technology based on the physical and psychological needs of those who use them.
    c. The purpose is to evaluate patient safety in healthcare organizations and identify the underlying causes of sentinel and near-miss events, and then develop safeguards to prevent the recurrence of the incidents.
    d. They use a quality approach to better understand and prevent future and ongoing threats to patient safety.

20. Which of the following best describes what occurs during the norming phase of Tuckman's model for team development?
    a. When the projects comes to a close and the team moves on, appreciating and reflecting on their growth as a team
    b. Selecting the team members based on the areas of expertise necessary to achieve optimal results
    c. Diffusing or quieting the naturally-occurring conflicts between different team members' communication style
    d. When team members are encouraged to assume responsibility for their assigned roles

21. In order to secure electronic files and reports, the clinician must do which of the following?
    a. Use computer screen locks and shortened time-out locks
    b. Use black-out screens whenever the computer is left unattended
    c. Limit access to computers
    d. All of the above

22. Root-cause analysis is used to do which of the following?
    a. Identify the cause of sentinel and near miss events
    b. Evaluate patient safety
    c. Answer the "why" questions
    d. All of the above

23. What is the purpose of the dashboard in performance improvement?
    a. Dashboards are tools that enable the management team to visually analyze the KPIs of each individual on the healthcare team.
    b. Dashboards depict the precipitating factors or root cause for an event or outcome
    c. Dashboards contain measurable data that indicates whether the goals and objectives are attainable.
    d. Dashboards are a written account that compares and measures the performance of individuals against the projected goals of the organization.

24. What are the two major stipulations of the Health Insurance Portability and Accountability Act of 1996?
    a. To protect the rights of healthcare organizations to deny medical care to indigent patients, and to prevent unnecessary malpractice suits
    b. To protect physicians' rights to provide medical care, and to hold healthcare organizations accountable for how patients' protected health information is utilized
    c. To protect patients against retaliation when reporting malpractice, and to hold healthcare organizations accountable for how patients' protected health information is utilized
    d. To protect patients' rights to maintain health-insurance coverage in the event of job loss, and to hold healthcare organizations accountable for how patients' protected health information is utilized

25. How frequently are scorecards used internally for performance improvement?
    a. Quarterly
    b. Quarterly and annually
    c. Annually
    d. Monthly and quarterly

26. What does the acronym NPS refer to?
    a. New Patient Safety
    b. National Patient Safety
    c. Net Promoter Score
    d. National Population Safety

27. The IHI Simple Data Collection Plan begins data collection planning by first doing which of the following?
    a. Asking why these data are being collected
    b. Deciding the tools to use
    c. Deciding on team members
    d. Setting goals

28. Which statement about near-miss and sentinel events is true?
    a. Both are ways to define an accident in a healthcare setting.
    b. Both events always prove that the provider was negligent in caring for the patient.
    c. A near-miss event does not result in death, while a sentinel event may result in death.
    d. The responsible party should always contact the police immediately.

29. What is the purpose of the cost-benefit analysis in process improvement?
    a. To determine the true costs of a potential solution compared to the actual benefits
    b. To ensure that the outcome actually solves the problem
    c. To confirm the passive and unplanned spread of new practices
    d. To find solutions before they become necessary

30. The Institute for Healthcare Improvement reported the six aims necessary to improve the current quality of healthcare as:
    a. safe, effective, problem-focused, timely, efficient, equitable
    b. secure, effective, patient-focused, timely, efficient, equitable
    c. satisfaction, expectancy, problem-focused, timeliness, efficiency, and eagerness
    d. safe, effective, patient-focused, timely, efficient, equitable

31. What do process measures show?
   a. If the team met their goals
   b. How the steps in the system perform
   c. If the measures improved care
   d. All of the above

32. Which of the following is true about FMEA?
   a. It is a program evaluation method that is primarily process based.
   b. It is a program evaluation method that is primarily outcome based.
   c. It is a program evaluation method that is primarily observation based
   d. It is a program evaluation method that is mandated by OSHA.

33. What is the advantage of identifying process champions for process and performance improvement projects?
   a. Process champions provide a visual representation of the current processes, in an effort to find areas of redundancy and lacking in value to the customer.
   b. It will always be more advantageous to consider the importance of adding to, rather than detracting from, the value delivered to customers.
   c. Process champions can identify potential pitfalls during the brainstorming phase of process improvement.
   d. Process champions ensure that the VOC is heard and to confirm that there is a precisely defined focus on the correct processes.

34. Internal benchmarking can be described as which of the following?
   a. Comparing similar processes to a competitor within the same industry
   b. Comparing equivalent processes within the same organization
   c. Comparing the general concepts of processes in unrelated industries
   d. Comparing similar processes to those in different industries

35. What is a process champion?
   a. An administrative team member
   b. Someone that has authority over the involved process
   c. A member of the process improvement team
   d. All of the above

36. What do control charts tell the team?
   a. The control limit of the process
   b. What processes are out of control
   c. If they met their goals
   d. How a process changes over time

37. The need for more extensive medical record keeping increased during what time period?
   a. 1950s
   b. 1960s
   c. 1970s
   d. 1980s

38. The core portions of the SIPOC method include which of the following?
    a. Suppliers, inputs, processes, outputs, customers
    b. Scorecards, inputs, processes, outputs, customers
    c. Sponsors, investors, products, outputs, customers
    d. Suppliers, inputs, processes, opportunities, consumers

39. Innovation in healthcare can best be described as which of the following?
    a. Passively spreading a new process or spreading it in an unplanned fashion
    b. A form of predictive technology that will enhance physicians' ability to provide medical care
    c. Developing a new process, policy, or standard that improves upon the quality outcomes of previous processes
    d. Providing a format to create uniformity of practice across other departments within the organization

40. What does a trend analysis help the team do best?
    a. Decide which trend to follow
    b. Understand historical data about a process
    c. Identify the mean, median, and mode
    d. Prove a hypothesis

41. Which of the following is true of telemedicine?
    a. It is a form of medical care provided remotely by credentialed and licensed healthcare professionals.
    b. It is prohibited by the Health Insurance Portability and Accountability Act of 1996.
    c. The primary role of the CPHQ professional.
    d. It is required by the Health Insurance Portability and Accountability Act of 1996.

42. What is the goal of the improve phase of the DMAIC model?
    a. To enable the management team to visually analyze the KPIs of each individual on the healthcare team
    b. To assimilate all the ideas into a strategic plan that prioritizes opportunities for improvement and amends all processes associated with changes, including any process flows and job aids
    c. During the improve phase of the DMAIC model, the CPHQ professional will need to implement strategies to determine the sustainability and benefits of the newly defined processes.
    d. During this phase, the manager enables team members to do it themselves.

43. What is the best description of a correlation?
    a. A correlation is a dependent relationship between two quantitative continuous variables and can either be positive or negative.
    b. A correlation is a way of using a selected group of individuals to rapidly produce, clarify, and evaluate ideas or problems.
    c. A correlation is an independent relationship between two quantitative continuous variables and can either be positive or negative.
    d. A correlation is defined as the continual and collaborative discipline of measuring and comparing the results of key work processes.

44. What is the VOB?
    a. The reputation of the business
    b. The needs of the business
    c. The organization's goals
    d. All of the above

45. Which of the following is true of competitive benchmarking?
    a. It is not advised by TJC.
    b. It can be done by reviewing the public summary on a competitor's website.
    c. It helps improve internal quality processes.
    d. It is not necessary for accreditation.

46. The most problematic issues of the EHR are caused by which of the following?
    a. Security measures
    b. Cyber crimes
    c. Human errors
    d. Passwords

47. Broken down into each individual function, what does the acronym DMAIC stands for?
    a. Define, measure, analyze, improve, control
    b. Define, measure, adjust, improve, complete
    c. Define, measure, amend, institute, control
    d. Depict, measure, analyze, improve, control

48. Which quality control tool is best suited to use when investigating short-term process improvement activities?
    a. Run charts
    b. T-tests
    c. Control charts
    d. Pareto charts

49. The HCAHPS initiative's goal is to provide a standardized survey instrument and data collection methodology for measuring which of the following?
    a. The quality of care in hospitals
    b. Patient satisfaction
    c. Employee satisfaction
    d. Patient perceptions of care

50. Extra safety and security measures are important for which specialized hospital area?
    a. ICU
    b. ED
    c. Surgery
    d. Nursery

51. What does the project charter typically include?
    a. The sponsor or the project, a champion or resource allocation manager, subject matter expert, process owner, process operator
    b. The primary reason for the project, the goal, the scope of the project, the budget and roles of each team member
    c. Yellow belt, green belt, black belt, master black belt, process champion, executives.
    d. Suppliers of inputs, materials to input, processes that convert inputs to outputs, outputs to provide to customers, customers

52. What is the suggested preparatory schedule for accreditation?
    a. Six months of current-process analysis in advance of survey
    b. One year of current-process analysis prior to survey
    c. At least one year of current-process analysis followed by status updates every three months
    d. It should begin preparing for the next survey immediately after this one ends

53. What does the acronym DMAIC refer to in the Lean Six Sigma project management model?
    a. Describe, manage, accountability, interpret, and compare
    b. Define, manage, analyze, interpret, and control
    c. Describe, measure, analyze, improve, and compare
    d. Define, measure, analyze, improve, and control

54. Any deviation from the standard process typically results in higher risk, according to which methodology?
    a. 5 S
    b. Six Sigma
    c. Lean
    d. National Safety Standards

55. Why is it important to review scorecards and dashboards during performance improvement projects?
    a. The professional accountability and adherence to ongoing performance and process improvement measures afford the chosen organization the opportunity to remain competitive in the healthcare marketplace.
    b. Managers must always remain diligent and keenly aware that the responses of the process innovators, early adopters, and the early majority will most likely determine the success of the newly developed process and performance expectation.
    c. The results from the aggregated quality and performance data equip the management team to develop specific, measurable, achievable, relevant, and timely (SMART) metrics for gauging the staff's effectiveness and efficiency.
    d. When employees feel that their contribution is linked to the mission, values, and goals of the host organization, they are more likely to accept responsibility for their results.

56. When meetings have dysfunctions, they impact which of the following?
    a. The quality agenda
    b. The cost and team confidence
    c. The cost, schedule, quality, and project manager's credibility
    d. The schedule and cost

57. A facilitator needs to consider all EXCEPT which of the following?
    a. The time available for meetings
    b. The structure of the meeting
    c. Which goals to set
    d. The number of team members

58. Which statement best describes the purpose of bundled payments?
    a. This initiative was established to encourage payers to employ a set of core measures to utilize during reporting.
    b. The primary goal is to produce more effective processes, policies, and procedures that reduce variation and significantly lower the chances of negative outcomes.
    c. This initiative depicts the active spread of those new practices to a target audience, utilizing planned methodologies.
    d. This initiative can best be defined as measurable data that will further indicate if the goals and objectives of the project are attainable.

59. What do Pareto charts allow the leadership team to do?
    a. Focus on the value of the services provided
    b. Focus on the just-in-time process timeline
    c. View statistics on their dashboard
    d. All of the above

60. Loyalty in adversity and an outcome-focused approach are 2 of the 5 factors of which of the following?
    a. Human Factor Engineering
    b. Standard Operating Procedures
    c. Lean/Six Sigma
    d. A high reliability organization

61. Why is it crucial to consider the voice of the customer (VOC) during process improvement?
    a. The customer's voice is the outward image of the business, and the reputation that the business has earned among consumers.
    b. The voice of the customer uses a selected group of individuals to rapidly produce, clarify, and evaluate ideas or problems.
    c. The customer's voice enables the leadership team to understand the passive and unplanned spread of new practices.
    d. During this phase, the manager can begin to take a less direct role and delegate activities to team members.

62. According to the Lean Six Sigma framework, which two quality tools are typically utilized in the analyze phase?
    a. Run charts and Pareto charts
    b. Process capability assessments and critical to quality trees
    c. Project charter and process mapping
    d. Brainstorming and benchmarking

63. Functions of the leadership team include which of the following?
    a. To ensure cohesion, define vision and values, ensure alignment, and deliver results
    b. To engage stakeholders, develop talent, and manage performance
    c. To build accountability, ensure succession, allocate resources and craft the culture
    d. All of the above

64. Why should correlations be reviewed with caution during process and performance improvement projects?
    a. At this stage, it is crucial to create linkages between the mission, goals, and objectives of the host organization to the actual performance metrics, skills, and quality standards of the supportive team members.
    b. The CPHQ professional will need to implement strategies to determine the sustainability and benefits of the newly defined processes.
    c. When considering what may go wrong, the team professional must determine whether the individual actions in the newly developed processes are logical.
    d. The team must remain aware that the data may only represent the relationship between variables, not the actual causes and effects of current processes.

65. Risk Managers are trained to evaluate which of the following?
    a. Potential for harm
    b. Outcomes of events
    c. Patient safety
    d. All of the above

66. What is values-based leadership?
    a. An attitude about people, philosophy, and process
    b. Leading by example rather than manipulation
    c. Integrity, listening, and respect for followers
    d. Clear thinking, inclusion, and respect

67. Which of the following is necessary for a team meeting to be considered successful?
    a. Actions have follow-up
    b. There are clear activities
    c. Process owners are present
    d. All of the above

68. What is the best description of positive correlation depicted in a scattergram?
    a. One variable decreases while another increases; the points on the scatter plot will be close together and trend up to the left in the form of a line.
    b. The correlation would yield a value of zero, with the data on the scatter plot appearing to have no clear shape or direction within the middle of the axes.
    c. One variable increases while another increases; the points on the scatter plot will be close together and trend up to the right in the form of a line.
    d. One variable increases while another increases, up to a certain point; the data points will resemble a checkmark.

69. What is the best definition of verification?
    a. The active spread of those new practices to a target audience utilizing planned methodologies
    b. A process that ensures that the outcome actually solves the problem.
    c. The testing that the proposed solution produces the desired outcome.
    d. Measurable data that will further indicate whether the goals and objectives are attainable.

70. What are organic organizations?

    I. Those that have a loose structure with more innovation and less specialization
    II. Those that have expertise and knowledge rather than authority of position
    III. Those that have loosely-defined responsibilities rather than rigid job definitions
    IV. Those with fewer constraints on the activity of members, enabling and encouraging the expression of individual behavior by leaders and potential followers

    a. Choices *I* and IV
    b. Choices III and IV
    c. Choices *I*, III, and IV
    d. All of the above

71. Which of the following best describes the Healthcare Effectiveness Data and Information Set (HEDIS)?
    a. The continual and collaborative discipline of measuring and comparing the results of key work processes
    b. A group of performance standards that the majority of health plans adhered to in an effort to standardize the overall quality of care delivered to patients
    c. The written agreement that acts as measurable data to indicate if the goals and objectives of the project are attainable
    d. The primary goal is to produce more effective processes, policies, and procedures that reduce variation and significantly lower the chances of negative outcomes

72. Which of the following is true regarding critical to quality measures?
    a. They are defined by the leadership team
    b. They are set by CMS
    c. They must be met to satisfy the customer
    d. They are always key processes

73. Systems thinking uses which of the following?
    a. A centrist approach
    b. Cognitive mapping
    c. Scorecards
    d. Technology to drive ideas

74. What are the two phases of the strategic quality planning process?
    a. Planning and implementing
    b. Research and implementing
    c. Strategy and implementing
    d. Research and strategy

75. What happens when the needs of the business do not meet the needs of the customer?
    a. Resources are exhausted
    b. Processes are improved
    c. Voice of the customer is needed
    d. Certification is not possible

76. Which Lean Six Sigma format targets current processes?
    a. Define, measure, analyze, improve, and control
    b. Define, maintain, analyze, improve, and control
    c. Define, measure, analyze, design, and verify
    d. Define, measure, analyze, investigate, and contain

77. What is the best description of statistical process control?
    a. The continual and collaborative discipline of measuring and comparing the results of key work processes
    b. The process by which numerous small general factors result in a specific effect on a process
    c. The specific rare factors that can influence a process
    d. A strategy for instituting ongoing process improvement

78. A patient suspected of having TB would be placed under what type of infection control?
    a. Universal precautions
    b. Droplet precautions
    c. Airborne precautions
    d. Contact precautions

79. What is the order of the Lean Six Sigma certification belts according to rising expertise level?
    a. White, yellow, green, black, master black
    b. Black, white, yellow, green, master black
    c. Master black, green, yellow, black, white
    d. White, green, yellow, black, master black

80. What factors are the primary focus of human-factors engineering?
    a. Devices and technologies based on the physical and psychological needs of those who use them
    b. How to build technology through asking a series of "why" questions
    c. Reliance on practical experience, loyalty in adversity, and an outcome-focused approach
    d. Build technology through measurement, analysis, and improving current technology

81. Which agency mandated that hospitals designate a chief compliance officer to have the responsibility of operating and monitoring the compliance program, and who reports directly to the CEO and the governing body?
    a. TJC
    b. Medicare
    c. CMS
    d. OIG

82. What is the best description of critical to quality measures?
    a. This quality control tool helps to emphasize the frequency of the most impactful problems in order to allocate the appropriate amount of resources to rectify the problem.
    b. Critical to quality measures graphically represent the variation of values within a group; this format depicts the center, spread, and shape of the data.
    c. Critical to quality measures can be defined as the specific measurable facets of a process whose performance standards must be met to satisfy the customer.
    d. This tool helps the CPHQ professional to determine the purpose, roles, scope, and budget of the investigation.

83. The action plan should include which of the following?
    a. Missing capacities
    b. Signatures of all team members
    c. Who, what, when, where, why and how
    d. A list of primary problem areas

84. What are key performance indicators (KPI)?
    a. Goals for change
    b. What employee evaluations are measured against
    c. Measurable data about organizational goals
    d. Attainable goals

85. What is output?
    a. Tangible results
    b. Goods and services
    c. Under team control
    d. All of the above

86. In healthcare risk management, an action or inaction that could have resulted in nonlethal injury to a patient is known as which of the following?
    a. A sentinel event
    b. An incident
    c. A near-miss event
    d. A human factor

87. Which of the following best describes a whistleblower?
    a. An individual protected from retaliation under the law
    b. An identified person who has information of importance
    c. Someone who was recently fired from the organization
    d. All of the above

88. What are indicators?
    a. Linked to objectives
    b. Measurable
    c. Linked to quality
    d. All of the above

89. What is the best method of noting quantitative or qualitative data?
    A. Scorecards
    b. Check sheets
    c. Fishbone diagrams
    d. KPI

90. When does implementation occur?
    a. When the board members sign off on the project
    b. When everyone on the team agrees on the process
    c. When practices are adopted and integrated
    d. When the team finishes its work

91. Organizations that adopt which of the following methods of risk management achieve a high level of excellence because they focus on anticipating the best response to the worst-case scenario?
    a. High Reliability
    b. Six Sigma
    c. Systems thinking
    d. Human Factor Engineering

92. Which statistical quality tool would be the best choice to depict the center, spread, and shape of data?
    a. Histograms
    b. Run chart
    c. Control charts
    d. Fishbone diagram

93. What are the primary goals of the OSHA inspection?
    a. To provide a reference for surveyors to specify deficiencies within the organization being evaluated
    b. To protect the safety of patients and/or residents in healthcare organizations
    c. To provide healthcare to individuals that cannot afford health insurance
    d. To protect the safety of the employees of healthcare organizations

94. Which of the following is included in the PLAN stage of PDSA?
    a. Complete the action plan
    b. Develop the calendar
    c. Test the validity of the plan
    d. Identify possible interventions

95. What is the difference between common cause variation and special cause variation?
    a. Common cause variation is the process by which numerous small general factors result in a specific effect on a process; special cause variation refers to the specific rare factors that can influence a process
    b. Common cause variation is the process of comparing equivalent processes within the same organization; special cause variation refers to comparing similar processes to a competitor within the same industry
    c. Common cause variation can be defined as the passive and unplanned spread of new practices; special cause variation is defined as the active spread of those new practices to target audience utilizing planned methodologies
    d. Common cause variation is the process by which a single payment is made to cover the costs of the treatment provided for any given treatment; special cause variation refers to measurable data that will further indicate if the goals and objectives are attainable

96. What is the difference between accreditation and certification?
    a. Accreditation and certification are the same; both are typically granted to individuals, organizations, and facilities.
    b. Accreditation is typically granted to organizations and facilities, whereas certification is typically granted to individuals.
    c. Accreditation is typically based on the total billed for the number individuals a physician provides care for, whereas certification is typically based on the quality of care provided.
    d. Accreditation is typically granted to individuals, whereas certification is typically granted to organizations and facilities.

97. What is the best definition of validation?
    a. The rate at which newly disseminated innovations are adopted and implemented
    b. Developing the necessary countermeasures to solve any problems before they actually occur
    c. A dependent relationship between two quantitative continuous variables
    d. A process that ensures that the outcome actually solves the problem

98. Outcome measures tell the organization how the system impacts which of the following?
    a. The organizational goals and values
    b. HEDIS measures
    c. Accreditation measures
    d. Values of patients and others

99. Lean Six Sigma drives customer satisfaction and the bottom line by doing which of the following?
    a. Analyzing PDSA steps closely
    b. Using Pareto charts to track improvement
    c. Using competitive benchmarking
    d. Reducing variation and waste

100. Cognitive mapping is important in the systems thinking approach because it is a way to do which of the following?
    a. Visualize what happened during the incident
    b. Visualize otherwise unnoticeable connections
    c. Visualize what the patient was thinking
    d. Visualize what to do next

101. What is the industry-standard methodology for measuring and controlling quality during the manufacturing process in real time with pre-determined control limits called?
   a. Lean manufacturing
   b. Statistical Process Control (SPC)
   c. Variability Index
   d. Quality Control (QC)

102. Protected health information (PHI) includes which of the following?
   a. The patient's EHR
   b. Physician orders
   c. Medical bills
   d. All of the above

103. What is the best definition for key performance indicators (KPIs)?
   a. The provider of inputs into a business process
   b. Measurable data that indicates whether the goals and objectives are attainable
   c. Materials and resources needed to complete a business process
   d. The products or services resulting from inputs during the implementation of a process

104. What is the purpose of the "five why's" in a root-cause analysis?
   a. To sift through current policies and reveal causal factors within the control of the team
   b. To make sure patients understand what happened
   c. To prepare an incident report
   d. To communicate the cause to the leadership of the organization

105. Public reporting of the survey results is designed to do what?
   a. Create incentives for hospitals to improve their quality of care
   b. Enhance public accountability in health care
   c. Increase the transparency of the quality of hospital care
   d. All of the above

106. What are two steps where data mistakes happen most often?
   a. Entering and collating
   b. Saving and editing
   c. Downloading and importing
   d. All of the above

107. What is the best definition for mistake-proofing?
   a. The ways to determine whether there is a dependent relationship between two quantitative continuous variables, which is either positive or negative
   b. Using a selected group of individuals to rapidly produce, clarify, and evaluate ideas or problems
   c. Developing the necessary countermeasures to solve any problems before they actually occur
   d. The election and introduction of team members based on the areas of expertise necessary to achieve optimal results

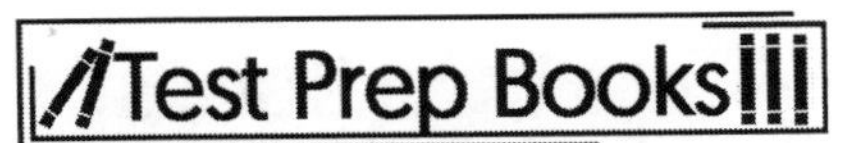

108. Why is it crucial for the leadership team to prepare the entire organization for the on-site survey portion of the accreditation process?

a. To actively observe any gaps in processes, procedures, and policies prior to the actual survey
b. To provide a uniformity of practice across other departments within the organization
c. To assure that the leadership team is prudent and acting in the best interests of the organization and in good faith
d. To encourage competition across other departments within the organization

109. What is the best definition of cost-benefit analysis?

a. Testing that the proposed solution produces the desired outcome
b. Quality measurement tools that actually enable the management team to visually analyze the KPIs of each individual on the healthcare team
c. The action or process of developing a new idea, methodology or action, that improves on its predecessor
d. An activity used in the Lean Six Sigma methodology as a way to determine the true costs of a potential solution compared to the actual benefits

110. Which of the following is true about non-probability sampling?

a. It is based on human choice
b. It uses volunteer samples
c. It contains sources of bias
d. All of the above

111. Which of the following are true regarding the Hospital Compare site?

I. It is free on the internet for everyone.
II. It communicates the CMS scores for every hospital in the U.S.
III. It posts the scores for healthcare quality measures.

a. Choices *I* and II
b. Choices *I* and III
c. Choices II and III
d. All of the above

112. What is the best definition of norming?

a. Norming is when people begin to resolve their differences and come to accept their coworkers' strengths.
b. Norming is a process that ensures that the outcome actually solves the problem.
c. Norming is the passive and unplanned spread of new practices.
d. Norming is measurable data that will further indicate whether the goals and objectives are attainable.

113. Why are peer reviews important for the maintenance of service quality and practitioner performance?

a. To help achieve and maintain full accreditation or certification
b. To prevent any legal violations or citations from accrediting bodies
c. To provide uniformity of practice across other departments within the organization
d. To allow colleagues to anonymously provide the constructive feedback necessary to guide performance-improvement initiatives

114. Which of these statements about failure mode and effect analysis is NOT true?
    a. Failure mode analysis is an outcome-based method of program evaluation.
    b. Failures are ranked in severity from one to five and managed in order of severity of three or greater.
    c. Analysts ask about the severity, probable cause, potential for harm, and patient detection.
    d. Failure mode analysts interview the patients involved in the incident.

115. What is the term for the tendency of a statistic to overestimate or underestimate a parameter?
    a. Central tendency
    b. Bias
    c. Smoothing
    d. Common cause variation

116. Why is it important to identify and report errors to regulatory and accrediting bodies?
    a. To create an atmosphere of patient-centered care within the organization
    b. To maintain ongoing accreditation
    c. To prevent any sanctions or violations for the organization
    d. To identify the appropriate employees to be held accountable

117. Which of the following best describes the purpose of storming?
    a. To develop countermeasures to solve any problems before they actually occur
    b. To explain the stages of the process and confirm that each team member is aware of their expected contribution
    c. To adopt and integrate practices in the proposed setting
    d. To visually analyze the KPIs of each individual on the healthcare team

118. What is a sentinel event?
    a. A method showing how 80% of the process efforts occur as a result of 20% of the causes
    b. An unforeseen occurrence that results in harm or death to a patient or group of patients
    c. All of the medical services for one individual patient for a specific medical condition
    d. An action or inaction that nearly resulted in a nonlethal injury to a patient

119. Which of the following is true regarding informed consent forms?
    a. They must be completed at admission
    b. They must be signed, dated, and witnessed
    c. They must be maintained under lock and key
    d. All of the above

120. With Tuckman's model (forming, storming, norming, performing) what is the primary goal of the forming stage?
    a. To encourage discussion among colleagues
    b. To form a strong team
    c. To meet the goals of the organization
    d. For the team to follow the facilitator's plan

121. What are the four types of benchmarking?
   a. Investigative, internal, external, and generic
   b. Internal, cooperative, external, and competitive
   c. Internal, competitive, functional, and generic
   d. Intensive, competitive, functional, and generic

122. Root-cause analysis is used to do which of the following?
   a. Analyze healthcare systems
   b. Prevent incidents from happening again
   c. Respond to OSHA complaints
   d. Investigate patients

123. What is diffusion?
   a. A method of brainstorming
   b. A way to control a team that is off course
   c. The passive spread of a new process
   d. Prohibited by most organizations

124. What is the best description of brainstorming?
   a. Brainstorming is defined as the continual and collaborative discipline of measuring and comparing the results of key work processes.
   b. Brainstorming can be referred to as a written account that compares and measures the performance of specific individuals against the projected goals of the organization.
   c. Brainstorming can best be defined as the rate at which newly disseminated ideas or innovations are adopted and implemented.
   d. Brainstorming can be referred to as a way of using a selected group of individuals to rapidly produce, clarify, and evaluate ideas or problems.

125. Every quality management initiative must be tied to what?
   a. The key business processes
   b. The mission and values
   c. How the competitors are doing
   d. Patient care

# Answer Explanations #1

**1. B:** If the answers regarding the issues addressed in a preliminary denial are provided by the organization to the TJC within 10 working days, the TJC will grant the accreditation so long as the answers are acceptable.

**2. C:** The primary goal of Lean Six Sigma is to produce more effective processes, policies, and procedures that reduce variation and significantly lower the chances of negative outcomes.

**3. D:** Critical to quality measures (CTQs) are the aspects of a business process or product that must be met in order to satisfy the consumer. This leads to a discovery of the voice of the customer (VOC), which is also crucial to improving processes.

**4. C:** The primary goal of The Joint Commission's adoption of the NPSGs is to encourage healthcare organizations to institute high quality standards for patient safety. The Joint Commission does not force organizations to comply with regulatory standards; federal regulations require adherence for reimbursement of healthcare services.

**5. B:** The most necessary step in evaluating the success of process improvement is executing the pilot study. The other choices do not evaluate the success of a PIP.

**6. B:** The project charter is a written agreement that usually includes that primary reason for the project, the goal and scope of the project, and the expected budget and roles of each member of the team.

**7. C:** During strategic planning, leadership's main task is to help the team understand the existing strategies and work to develop new ones that align with and support corporate goals.

**8. C:** Before sending out a meeting invite, the most important thing is that the facilitator must define the objectives of the meeting. They should also establish the tangible outcomes or outputs that the team aims to achieve. Doing so sets expectations and will ensure that people know precisely what is expected.

**9. A:** Choice *A* is correct; SIPOC stands for suppliers, inputs, processes, outputs, customers.

**10. C:** The incident report is reviewed first in most healthcare risk management assessments. Recall that the three main principles of risk management assessment are risk assessment, risk avoidance, and risk control. In the most critical step, risk assessment, what happened and why is considered. The analyst will need access to all available records, participants, policies, and procedures associated with the event. Methodical and purposeful deconstruction of every step should be mapped, and any discrepancies in processes, hardware, human factors, and organizational culture scrutinized. Similar incidents and associated resolutions within other healthcare settings should be compared and analyzed for probability of success.

**11. A:** The fiduciary duty-to-care regulation involves assurances that the board members are acting in good faith, in a prudent and reasonable fashion, and making decisions that are in the best interests of the organization. This rule essentially provides the board time to prepare a prompt response or adjust any detected errors or concerns.

**12. B:** Using scorecards and dashboards during a performance review can help highlight areas where additional training around related processes and procedures is needed. Choice *A* is incorrect because it

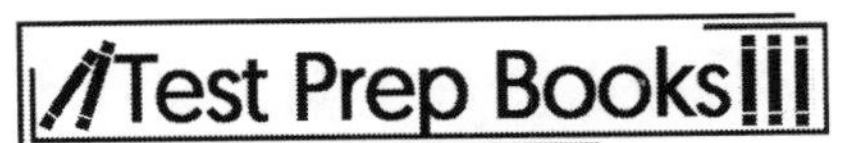

describes the purpose of process mapping. Choice *C* is incorrect because it describes the forming step of Tuckman's model. Choice *D* is an aspect of effective team communication, so it is incorrect.

**13. A:** Credentialing involves the oversight of licensing to medical professionals under their scope of practice, which means assessing their education, certifications, and training. Privileging refers to the evaluation of a practitioner's actual performance and qualifications, and includes granting practitioners benefits based on their abilities.

**14. C:** Scorecards can be defined as a written account that compares and measures the performance of specific individuals against the projected goals of the organization; dashboards are quality measurement tools that actually allow the management team to compare and contrast different reports or access diverse datasets in one place. They visually present summaries, key trends, comparisons, and exceptions.

**15. C:** Raw performance data is taken directly from the occurrence of tasks in the process flow. The other choices provided are incorrect descriptions. Choice *A* describes a project charter, Choice *B* describes KPIs, and Choice *D* describes correlation.

**16. D:** Data management involves acquiring, validating, storing, protecting, and processing data. The other choices are incorrect because data management procedures are a responsibility of personnel at all levels, and are not restricted only to local servers or cloud services.

**17. A:** Processes should be evaluated frequently to eliminate waste and reduce risk. Choice *B* is incorrect; The Joint Commission does not explicitly mandate frequent evaluations, but rather they should be done to meet accreditation requirements. Choices *C* and *D* are incorrect because, although they might reinforce employee training and reevaluate their effectiveness, the main purpose is reducing waste, redundancy, and risk.

**18. C:** Engaging department leaders, top performers, risk-management staff, and the medical governing board in discussions regarding how each department has succeeded in its adherence to the organization's mission, values, and strategic goals is one of the best ways to prepare for a survey.

**19. A:** The majority of policies and procedures enacted by healthcare organizations to ensure patient safety include factors that meet The Joint Commission's requirements and National Patient Safety goals.

**20. D:** Tuckman's model of team building includes five steps: forming, storming, norming, performing, and adjourning. Norming occurs after storming. In this stage, members are encouraged to assume responsibility for their assigned roles, and they come to recognize each other's strengths and resolve their differences. Managers play the pivotal role of acts as scaffolding, keeping the team members on task and fostering more collaboration. Choice *A* describes adjourning. Choice *B* describes forming. Choice *C* describes storming.

**21. D:** In order to secure electronic files and reports, the clinician must use computer screen locks and shortened time-out locks, use black-out screens whenever the computer is left unattended, and limit access to computers.

**22. D:** All of the above. The root-cause analysis is used to evaluate patient safety in healthcare environments. It identifies the cause of sentinel and near-miss events by asking "why" questions regarding the incident with the goal of process improvement.

**23. A:** Dashboards are quality measurement tools that enable the management team to visually analyze the KPIs of each individual on the healthcare team. Choice *B* is incorrect since it describes the role of a fishbone diagram. Choice *C* is related, since it describes the purpose of KPIs, but the question asks for the purpose of dashboards, so it is incorrect. Choice *D* describes the role of scorecards.

**24. D:** The two major stipulations of the Health Insurance Portability and Accountability Act of 1996 are to protect patients' rights to maintain health-insurance coverage in the event of job loss, and to hold healthcare organizations accountable for how patients' protected health information is utilized.

**25. B:** Scorecards are used internally during quarterly and annual employee evaluations. The other choices represent intervals that are too often or too infrequent.

**26. B:** NPS is the acronym for National Patient Safety. The Joint Commission established the NPS goals in 2002 and implemented them in 2003. This nationwide effort instituted a set of uniform, realistic, and specific goals that could be consistently applied and measured in every healthcare setting. National Patient Safety goals are set annually and have established the standard for excellence.

**27. A:** The IHI Simple Data Collection Plan begins data collection planning by first asking why data are being collected. Additional questions to consider include things like what type of data will be necessary, what data analysis tools will be used to display that obtained data, and where and how the data can be obtained.

**28. C:** A near-miss event does not result in death, while a sentinel event may result in death. Choice *A* is incorrect because a near-miss event is an avoided incident. Choice *B* is incorrect because a near-miss event is not necessarily a result of negligence, and may be the result of unforeseeable circumstances. Choice *D* is incorrect because such events are instead reported to The Joint Commission.

**29. A:** This is an activity used in the Lean Six Sigma methodology as a way to determine the true costs of a potential solution, as compared to the actual benefits.

**30. D:** The IHI aims to make healthcare safe, effective, patient-focused, timely, efficient, and equitable.

**31. B:** Process measures show the steps in the system perform. They are used to indicate to consumers what a healthcare provider will do to maintain or improve health.

**32. B:** Failure mode and effect analysis (FMEA) is a program evaluation method that is primarily outcome based. It seeks to uncover ways that business leaders can most effectively operationalize the efforts of frontline staff.

**33. C:** Process champions can identify potential pitfalls during the brainstorming phase of process improvement. These individuals are team members with the administrative authority to allocate time and resources for a project.

**34. B:** Internal benchmarking involves examining processes in different departments and teams within the same company or organization to determine best practices for the organization as a whole.

**35. D:** A process champion is an administrative leader who is a team member with the authority to allocate the time and resources needed to plan and launch the program. The process champion should also have authority over the areas that will be affected by changes to clinical and administrative systems and practices; and coordinate communication internally to senior leadership, Board of Directors, staff,

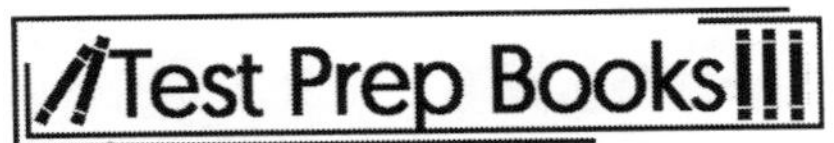

etc. They provide positive action-oriented leadership to ensure that process improvement projects get across the goal line.

**36. D:** Control charts show a process changes over time. As line graphs, they clearly indicate trends and patterns of specific processes, and how well that process is performing.

**37. C:** The 1970s ushered in a need for more extensive medical record keeping. With the influx of American veterans returning home needing significant medical and psychiatric care, paper medical files were largely traded in for computerized records.

**38. A:** SIPOC stands for suppliers, inputs, processes, outputs, and customers. It is a process improvement tool used to define each step of a process before it's implemented.

**39. C:** Innovation involves developing a new process, policy, or standard that improves upon the quality outcomes of previous processes. Choice *A* refers to diffusion. Choice *B* refers to patient analytics and medical informatics. Choice *D* refers to internal benchmarking.

**40. B:** A trend analysis helps the team understand historical data about a process. Choice *A* is incorrect because the analysis observes past trends to understand why they occurred. Choice *C is* wrong because identifying the mean, median, and mode of a data set is only one aspect of identifying trends. While trend analysis may be useful in disproving a hypothesis, one cannot prove a hypothesis true, so Choice *D* is incorrect.

**41. A:** Telemedicine is a form of medical care provided remotely by credentialed and licensed healthcare professionals. It has reformed healthcare delivery across the country. Providers can now conduct patient assessments, prescribe medications, and collaborate with other medical professionals remotely, via Skype, telephone, email, and secure chatrooms. This type of distance healthcare eliminates the constraints of geography and mobility, and allows providers access to increasing numbers of previously underserved populations.

**42. B:** The goal is to assimilate all the ideas into a strategic plan that prioritizes opportunities for improvement and amends all processes associated with changes, including any process flows and job aids.

**43. A:** A correlation is a dependent relationship between two quantitative continuous variables and can either be positive or negative. Choice *B* is incorrect because it describes brainstorming. Choice *C* is incorrect because a correlation is found between dependent, not independent, variables. Choice *D* describes benchmarking, so it is also incorrect.

**44. B:** The voice of the business (VOB) includes the implicit and explicit needs and requirements of the business, such as profit, competitive edge, and growth. It is an important process measure for meeting the business's goals.

**45. B:** Competitive benchmarking can help reveal how similar organizations solved defects similar to what a given healthcare organization is facing. The comparative analysis can also illuminate how the current processes are outpacing the competitors, which encourages the integration of what works with what does not work well enough. This approach will help the leadership team to deliver on the promise of providing exceptional care. All hospitals have to post their quality information on their websites for the public view.

**46. C:** One pitfall of the electronic medical record involves the human factor. Since a computer is only capable of providing information based on what is entered, information entered inaccurately or omitted has the potential to harm a patient.

**47. A:** The DMAIC acronym stands for define, measure, analyze, improve, control. This is an important tool in the Six Sigma model of process improvement.

**48. A:** Run charts are best suited to investigate short-term process improvement activities. Like control charts, they are line graphs that indicate trends and patterns of specific processes, and how well that process is performing.

**49. D:** The Hospital Consumer Assessment of Healthcare Providers and Systems (HCAHPS) initiative's goal is to provide a standardized survey instrument and data collection methodology for measuring patient perceptions of care. This allows patients to compare hospitals' quality of care (in multiple areas) based on the survey scores from other patients.

**50. D:** Nursery. Due to the possibility of an abduction, there are special safeguards in place.

**51. B:** The project charter includes the primary reason for the project, the goal, the scope of the project, the budget, and the roles of each team member. The project charter is not a list of individuals involved in the project, so Choices *A* and *C* are incorrect. Choice *D* is incorrect because it describes the steps of SIPOC, not the purpose of a project charter.

**52. C:** The suggested preparatory schedule for accreditation typically involves a year of planning along with close monitoring. The other choices represent incorrect timelines for planning.

**53. D:** DMAIC stands for define, measure, analyze, improve, and control. The DMAIC model helps improve existing processes and allows for the methodical development of an action plan to streamline and standardize laborious processes, reduce waste, and mitigate risks to the patient population in any healthcare setting.

**54. B:** According to Six Sigma, any deviation from the standard process typically results in higher risk. Choice *A,* the 5 S method, is incorrect because it is an organization tool used in Lean. Choice *C,* Lean, is incorrect because it focuses specifically on reducing waste, not variety. The National Safety Standards are not a methodology in process improvement, so Choice *D* is incorrect.

**55. C:** The results from the aggregated quality and performance data equip the management team to develop specific, measurable, achievable, relevant, and timely (SMART) metrics for gauging the staff's effectiveness and efficiency.

**56. C:** Meeting dysfunctions have significant negative impacts on the progress of the project. Dysfunctional meetings impact the cost, schedule, and quality of the project, but also reduce the project manager's credibility within the team.

**57. C:** Goals are set by the team during the meeting, not solely by the facilitator. The allowed time, meeting structure, and members in the meeting are all responsibilities of the facilitator.

**58. A:** Bundled payments were established to encourage payers to employ a set of core measures to utilize during reporting. Choice *B* is incorrect because it describes the purpose of Lean Six Sigma. Choice

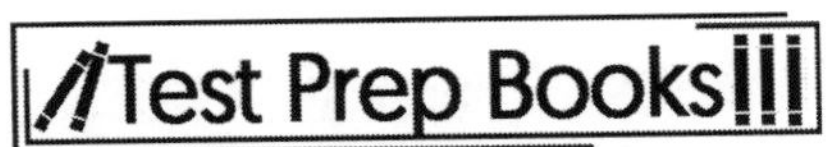

*C* is incorrect because it describes dissemination. Choice *D* describes the key performance indicators, not bundled payments, so it is incorrect.

**59. A:** Pareto charts track key operations over time, allowing leadership to identify the most significant issues affecting quality. Pareto charts are not related to the just-in-time training process and are only one component of quality statistics.

**60. D:** Loyalty in adversity and an outcome-focused approach are 2 of the 5 factors in any high-reliability organization. The other three are reliance on practical experience, an emphasis on operationalized definitions of expected outcomes, and a deeper-dive perspective when unexpected problems arise. Organizations that adopt this method of risk management achieve a high level of excellence because they focus on anticipating the best response to the worst-case scenario.

**61. A:** The customer's voice is the outward image of the business, and the reputation that the business has earned among consumers. Understanding the VOC is critical for developing processes and products that are customer-focused.

**62. A:** The run and Pareto charts are most frequently used in the analyze stage. Choice *B* is incorrect because the terms describe measurements used to determine a process's success and are not a key component of the DMAIC analyze phase. Choice *C* is incorrect because a project charter is used to outline the stages of a project, while process mapping involves diagramming the steps of a process. The tools in Choice *D* are used to improve processes through new ideas.

**63. D:** Leadership teams have many roles. They should strive to do all of the things listed here.

**64. D:** The team must remain aware that the data may only represent the relationship between variables, not the actual causes and effects of current processes. The other choices do not represent reasons for caution when reviewing correlations.

**65. D:** Risk managers are trained in many things including the potential for harm, outcomes of events, and patient safety.

**66. A:** Values-based leadership is based on an attitude of the value of people, processes and philosophy. The other choices represent parts of values-based leadership, but do not describe it as a whole.

**67. D:** For a team meeting to be successful, actions must have follow-up, there must be clear activities, and process owners must be present. A beneficial meeting is one that generates follow-up, and in order to best generate that follow-up, the meeting must define the process owners, review dates, and have clear actions to take.

**68. C:** A positive correlation occurs when one variable increases while another increases; the points on the scatterplot will be close together and trend up to the right in the form of a line. The other choices represent different types of correlations. A negative correlation would show one variable decreasing while the other increases and trend up to the left. No correlation in a scatterplot would present data not fitting close to any line, while a curvilinear correlation corresponds to data points that fit best to a non-linear shape, such as a checkmark or parabola.

**69. C:** Verification refers to testing that the proposed solution produces the desired outcome. Choice *A* is incorrect because it describes diffusion. Choice *B* describes validation, so it is incorrect. Choice *D* is incorrect because it describes KPIs.

**70. D:** Organic organizations are relatively flexible and adaptive and have a loose structure that is appropriate for changing conditions. They emphasize lateral communication and exchanging information rather than the vertical handing down of instructions. Organic organizations tend to be more innovative and less specialized. They utilize experts and knowledge rather than position authority. They offer loose responsibilities rather than rigid job descriptions. Their decentralized decision-making processes, are less standardized and the division of labor is less structured. Additionally, they impose fewer constraints on the activity of members and they encourage the expression of individual behavior.

**71. B:** The Healthcare Effectiveness Data and Information Set (HEDIS) is a group of performance standards that the majority of health plans adhere to in an effort to standardize the overall quality of care delivered to patients. The other choices are incorrect; Choice *A* describes benchmarking, Choice *C* describes key performance indicators, and Choice *D* describes the main goal of Lean Six Sigma.

**72. C:** Critical to quality measures are the aspects of a business process or product that must be met in order to satisfy the consumer. These are used to help split up customer demands into distinct, prioritizable items to improve on.

**73. B:** Systems thinking uses cognitive mapping to represent physical locations. Reviewing areas where each department connects to others can help identify more points of interaction that contribute to incidents.

**74. D:** The strategic quality planning process consists of research and strategy. The research phase serves a preparatory phase, which involves everything necessary to collect and analyze data before the strategic quality planning starts. The strategy phase incorporates the steps needed to develop the actual plan. Every initiative must be tied to the key business processes and their performance indicators or there would be no real impact on the balance sheet.

**75. A:** When the needs of the business do not meet the needs of the customer, resources will be exhausted. This necessitates the use of needs assessment to find what organization goals aren't being met.

**76. A:** The Lean Six Sigma format that targets current processes is DMAIC, which stands for define, measure, analyze, improve, and control.

**77. D:** Statistical process control is a strategy for instituting ongoing process improvement. It is the industry-standard methodology for measuring and controlling quality during the manufacturing process in real time with pre-determined control limits.

**78. C:** Airborne precautions are used with patients suspected of having TB.

**79. A:** The correct level-by-level categorization of Lean Six Sigma certification is white, yellow, green, black, and master black. Each successive level of certification demands a higher level of proficiency in Six Sigma methodology.

**80. A:** Human-factors engineering, also known as ergonomics, is the discipline that develops devices and technology based on the physical and psychological needs of those who use them. This field combines technological advances in healthcare with the specific needs of humans in mind. Choice *B* is incorrect because series of "why" questions are used for determining root cause. Choice *C* describes the benefits of the High Reliability approach to risk management. Improving current technology is not the primary goal of human-factor engineering, so Choice *D* is incorrect.

**81. D:** The OIG mandated that hospitals designate a chief compliance officer to have the responsibility of operating and monitoring the compliance program, and who reports directly to the CEO and the governing body.

**82. C:** Critical to quality (CTQ) measures can be defined as the specific measurable facets of a process whose performance standards must be met to satisfy the customer. It is necessary to know CTQs in order to best identify problems.

**83. C:** The action plan should always include the who, what, when, where, why and how. The action plan includes a list of existing capacities in order to *identify* missing capacities, so Choice *A* is incorrect. Choice *B* is incorrect because responsible parties, not member signatures, are an aspect of action plans. Problem areas are not determined by the action plan, so Choice *D* is incorrect.

**84. C:** Key performance indicators (KPIs) are measurable data about organizational goals. KPIs are not goals, but rather the data that indicates whether goals can be met, so Choices *A* and *D* are incorrect. While KPIs may be used in evaluating employee productivity, KPIs represent data on the organization level, and are not always used to evaluate employees, thus Choice *B* is incorrect.

**85. D:** The outcome and outputs for each objective of an action plan have to be identified. While the outcome is the development outcome at the end of the NSDS implementation, or, more specifically, the expected benefits to the target groups, the outputs are the direct and tangible results (goods and services) that will be delivered. Outputs are largely under the project management control.

**86. C:** In healthcare risk management, an action or inaction that could have resulted in nonlethal injury to a patient is known as a near miss event. These must be reduced and eliminated as much as possible to promote safe, high-quality healthcare.

**87. A:** A whistleblower is protected under law. While the other choices may actually be true of whistleblowers in some situations, they are not always the case (nor are they ideal), leaving Choice *A* as the best choice.

**88. D:** Indicators are linked to objectives and quality and are measurable. These are an aspect of action plan frameworks and measure how the objectives, purpose, results, and activities will be achieved.

**89. B:** Check sheets are best for notating data for collection when data can be collected by the same person at the same time.

**90. C:** Implementation occurs when practices are adopted and integrated. This is one of the four aspects of starting a new process or method in an organization.

**91. A:** Organizations that adopt the High Reliability methods of risk management achieve a high level of excellence because they focus on anticipating the best response to the worst-case scenario. This model provides transparency, accountability, and shared responsibility within the organization that reinforces problem solving.

**92. A:** Histograms are the best format to depict the center, spread, and shape of aggregated data. Run and control charts focus on trends of process performance, while control charts additionally show control limits to visualize how close data is to the average or being an outlier. Fishbone diagrams instead are used to illustrate root causes of an outcome.

**93. D:** This answer is correct because it refers to the primary goal of an OSHA inspection.

**94. D:** The PLAN stage of the PDSA involves identifying a goal or purpose, formulating an intervention or theory for change, defining success metrics and putting a plan into action. When using PDSA to improve a process, the first step is to identify possible goals and strategies to implement. After the goal is set, it's necessary to identify possible interventions and select one that seems promising.

**95. A:** Common cause variation is the process by which numerous small general factors result in a specific effect on a process; special cause variation refers to the specific rare factors that can influence a process. Both types of cause variation represent events that contribute to waste and errors.

**96. B:** Accreditation is typically granted to organizations and facilities, whereas certification is typically granted to individuals.

**97. D:** Validation is a process that ensures that the outcome. This occurs after the verification stage of process evaluation. Choice *A* is incorrect; the rate at which newly disseminated innovations are adopted and implemented is the definition of spread. Choice *B* is incorrect because it refers to mistake-proofing, and Choice *D* is incorrect because it describes correlation.

**98. D:** Outcome measures tell the organization how the system impacts the values of patients and others. They reflect the impact of the health care service or intervention on the health status of patients served. While they may seem to represent the gold standard in measuring quality, an outcome is the result of numerous factors, many beyond providers' control.

**99. D:** Lean Six Sigma drives customer satisfaction and the bottom line by reducing variables and waste. The term comes from a combination of two methodologies. The Six Sigma methodology focuses on the standardization and reduction of variation, while Lean focuses on waste reduction.

**100. B:** Cognitive mapping in systems thinking is used to represent physical locations. Areas where each subsystem perceives its connections to others can help identify more points of interaction that contribute to incidents.

**101. B:** Statistical Process Control is the industry-standard methodology for measuring and controlling quality during the manufacturing process in real time with pre-determined control limits.

**102. D:** PHI includes all health information that might identify the patient. Everything in the patient's EHR, including physician orders and medical bills, is part of PHI.

**103. B:** Key performance indicators (KPIs) are the measurable data that indicate whether the goals and objectives are attainable. These are often developed from trends of past data.

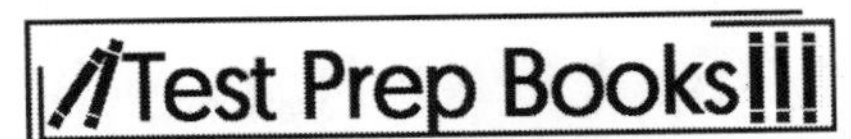

**104. A:** The "five why's" help sift through current policies and reveal causal factors within the control of the team. This process takes a problem and asks why the problem occurred, why the problem's most direct cause occurred, and so on, in order to determine the initial, or root, cause.

**105. D:** Transparency is the goal of public reporting of survey results because it can enhance public accountability in health care. Public reporting of the survey results also creates incentives for hospitals to improve their quality of care.

**106. C:** Downloading and importing are the two areas where most data mistakes occur. These steps should always be double checked to reduce errors.

**107. C:** Mistake-proofing develops countermeasures to solve problems before they occur. Once potential issues are identified, steps can be taken to prevent them. Choice *A* is irrelevant to mistake-proofing. Choice *B* describes brainstorming, so it is incorrect. Choice *D* is part of the forming step of the Tuckman model.

**108. A:** Preparatory training is the best way to get a close look at all areas of the organization before the survey.

**109. D:** The cost-benefit analysis is an activity used in the Lean Six Sigma methodology as a way to determine the true costs of a potential solution compared to the actual benefits. It is frequently necessary to conduct a cost-benefit analysis at the start of the project charter, during the define phase, and throughout implementation of the project.

**110. D:** Non-probability sampling should be avoided because it involves volunteer samples and haphazard (convenience) samples, which are based on human choice rather than random selection. Statistical theory cannot explain how the samples might behave and potential sources of bias are rampant.

**111. D:** In 2016 CMS unveiled the Overall Hospital Quality Star Ratings on its Hospital Compare website. The rating system combines 64 public measures into a single, one-to-five star rating. CMS rated more than 3,000 hospitals on the star scale. This website is free to the public.

**112. A:** Norming is when people begin to resolve their differences and come to accept their coworkers' strengths. This is the third stage in Tuckman's team-building model. Members are encouraged to assume responsibility for their assigned roles. The manager acts as scaffolding, keeping the team members on task and fostering more collaboration.

**113. D:** It is often necessary for colleagues to provide input regarding the performance of their coworkers to highlight strengths and weaknesses not readily observed by management.

**114. B:** It is not true that failures are ranked in severity from 1-5, and managed in order of severity over the rank of 3. They are ranked for 1-10, put in descending order, and those ranked at greater than 5 are managed in order of severity.

**115. B:** Bias is the tendency of a statistic to overestimate or underestimate a parameter. It can occur from sampling or measurement errors, or by using unrepresentative samples. If the statistic is unbiased, the average of all statistics from all samples will average the true population parameter.

**116. A:** Choice *A* is the best answer and clearly articulates why error reporting is significant. Choice *B* is incorrect because this is not the most important reason. Choice *C* is incorrect because sanctions are not automatically levied against an organization that reports errors. Choice *D* is incorrect because individual employees are protected against organizational retaliation when reporting errors; reporters remain anonymous.

**117. B:** The goal of storming is to explain the stages of the process and confirm that each team member is aware of their expected contribution. Storming is the second stage of Tuckman's model. In this step, mutual trust in the team is built as each team member begins to recognize their separate and collective strengths.

**118. B:** A sentinel event is an unforeseen occurrence that results in harm or death to a patient or group of patients. These events require immediate attention. Choice *A* is incorrect as it describes the 80-20 rule. Choice *C* describes an episode of care, so it is also incorrect. Choice *D* is incorrect because it describes a near-miss event, in which no injury actually occurs but might have, if not for intervention or fortune.

**119. D:** All of the choices are accurate statements regarding informed consent. Informed consent forms must be completed at admission. Additionally, they must be signed, dated, and witnessed, as well as maintained under lock and key (in the case of hard copies).

**120. A:** The goal of the forming stage of Tuckman's model is to encourage discussion among colleagues. Forming is the first step in Tuckman's model. During this stage, the team manager will choose members based on the areas of expertise necessary to achieve optimal results.

**121. C:** The four types of benchmarking are internal, competitive, functional, and generic. They allow the organization to measure and compare key work processes.

**122. B:** Root-cause analysis is a tool used to evaluate patient safety in healthcare organizations. The process identifies the underlying causes of sentinel and near-miss events and helps develop safeguards to prevent the recurrence of the incidents.

**123. C:** Diffusion is the passive and unplanned spread of new practices. Diffusion is said to occur through a five-step decision-making process culminating in the choice of whether or not to use a new idea.

**124. D:** Brainstorming can be referred to as a way of using a selected group of individuals to rapidly produce, clarify, and evaluate ideas or problems. Staff must be encouraged to preview the preliminary data, and leadership must allow for an open-ended and honest critique of what does and does not work.

**125. B:** Quality management initiatives should be tied to the mission and values of the organization to achieve sustainable change. Most organizational change is not maintained because it is not tied into the current culture or it is so different than the culture that employees do not embrace it. Issues that may negatively impact the sustainability of a project should be identified at both the planning and implementation stages.

# Practice Test #2

1. Which of the following choices is consistent with the definition of the strategic quality planning process?
   a. The strategy phase includes the analysis of data related to the proposed project.
   b. The research phase is associated with changes in the balance sheet.
   c. The overall strategic quality plan must be based on key performance indicators (KPIs).
   d. The process consists of three phases: research, strategy, and cost containment.

2. Which of the following activities is consistent with the process of data cleansing?
   a. Review the content of all datasets for unexpected findings.
   b. Merge datasets to capture novel data.
   c. Eliminate all visible documentation errors.
   d. Collect data from multiple sources.

3. According to the Eisenhower matrix, which of the following items is urgent and important?
   a. Planning an in-service activity for next year
   b. Moderating today's panel discussion for a colleague who is ill
   c. Reading an Instagram invitation to submit an abstract for a conference
   d. Re-organizing the email inbox

4. Which of the following describes the general characteristics of mechanistic organizations?
   a. Social change
   b. Centralized management
   c. Lateral communication
   d. Individual expression

5. What is the primary expected outcome when portions of the agenda are assigned to different individuals?
   a. Effective time management
   b. Presentation experience for additional team members
   c. Decreased workload for the facilitator
   d. Positive participant engagement

6. Which of the following choices is consistent with the data analysis e-measures developed by the NQF?
   a. The NQF reviews hospital use of e-measures every three years.
   b. Hospitals are required to use NQF e-measures for data reporting.
   c. CMS requires reporting on all 113 NQF measures.
   d. Hospitals can use the Measure Authoring Tool for measure development.

7. How does benchmarking affect the strategic quality planning process?
   a. It adds the voice of the customer.
   b. The resulting information dictates the new organizational strategy.
   c. It controls vendor pricing.
   d. Strategic planners learn from the experience of other organizations.

8. The facilitator is planning to use multivoting on a new list of possible solutions generated during a previous meeting. Which of the following techniques would be most helpful in this situation?
    a. The Eisenhower Matrix
    b. Small group discussion
    c. An affinity diagram
    d. Brainstorming session

9. The IHI data collection plan provides a framework for data collection for quality improvement efforts. Which of the following choices is consistent with that plan?
    a. The plan requires the generation of new data to identify areas for improvement.
    b. Sampling slows the process because large sample sizes are required for analysis.
    c. Useful data, rather than research-quality data, is required for a successful improvement plan.
    d. The cost of using data collection plans in individual hospitals generally exceeds the benefit.

10. The Agency for Healthcare Research and Quality (AHRQ) has published a survey to assess an agency's culture of safety. Which of the following areas would NOT be included in this assessment?
    a. Cost per patient admission
    b. Environmental service plan
    c. Patient portal usage
    d. Temporary staffing rates

11. Which of the following definitions is consistent with goal setting in the strategic quality planning process?
    a. Short-term goals are more appropriate in healthcare organizations.
    b. Organizational planners decide on the specific goals for the institution.
    c. Long-term goals are usually met successfully.
    d. Goals are set according to present circumstances.

12. Once a scribe has been assigned to assist with meeting details, the facilitator remains responsible for which of the following activities?
    a. Room accommodations
    b. Availability of appropriate IT resources
    c. Plans for follow-through of actions taken
    d. Attendance documentation as required for individual participants

13. Which of the following choices is NOT one of the four basic principles that guide institutional goal setting?
    a. Eliminate all inequalities.
    b. Strengthen information technology structures.
    c. Decrease provider workload.
    d. Encourage local improvement solutions.

14. The team leaders are assessing the time policy for ER-to-nursing-unit transfers. According to the IHI plan, which of the following sampling methods is most appropriate?
    a. Convenience sampling
    b. Block sampling
    c. Self-selection sampling
    d. Systematic sampling

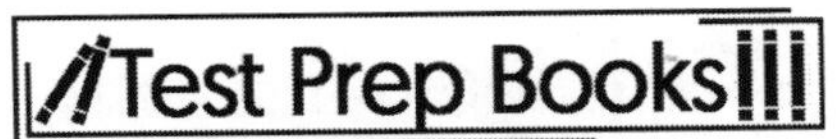


15. Which of the following choices describes the function of key performance indicators (KPIs)?
   a. Annual employee performance appraisal
   b. Long-range planning models for larger healthcare systems
   c. Measurement of growth potential for individual primary providers
   d. Measurable standards of performance that can reveal areas of weakness

16. Team leaders are estimating RN staffing requirements for the next fiscal year. Which of the following would be an appropriate outcome measure?
   a. Daily bed turnover rate
   b. Medication reconciliation
   c. Fall assessment
   d. Skin assessment

17. A team is reviewing institutional Critical to Quality Measures (CTQ measures). What is the relationship between these measures and institutional process improvement?
   a. CTQs are customer-based priorities
   b. CTQs are imposed by CMS
   c. CTQs are directly related to financial profit
   d. CTQs can replace KPIs (key performance indicators) in the planning process

18. Which of the following activities is an example of mistake proofing?
   a. Surgical "time out"
   b. Quiet environment rules
   c. Valet patient parking
   d. Patient portal appointment scheduling

19. According to recent research, the EHR (electronic health record) improves patient safety. Which of the following choices has been identified as a significant safety issue associated with its use?
   a. Inventory charges are not recorded.
   b. Computer access time is increased.
   c. Providers demonstrate alarm fatigue.
   d. Additional IT support is required.

20. Which of the following choices is consistent with the definition of diffusion?
   a. In-service educational modules for all certified nursing assistants
   b. Person-to-person discussion of possible changes
   c. Use of the new CAUTI (catheter-associated urinary tract infection) bundle
   d. Community vaccination information sessions

21. Which of the following choices is consistent with the stratified sampling method?
   a. The sampling for the patient satisfaction survey sample included males and females.
   b. The HbA1C level was measured for every sixth patient in the diabetic clinic population.
   c. Annual prostate exam rates were compared for two random groups of Medicare patients.
   d. Blood pressure readings were measured for volunteer employees.

22. When is a "time out" required?
    a. When AM medications are given
    b. Prior to lab testing for an infection
    c. Before the start of a colonoscopy
    d. When a chest x-ray is done

23. Which of the following choices would be an output for an action plan objective?
    a. Central line infection rates will be zero this quarter.
    b. RNs will complete a dressing change module.
    c. Nursing staff will demonstrate safe practice.
    d. Patient pain satisfaction scores will increase

24. Which of the following choices is consistent with the Centers for Medicare & Medicaid Services (CMS)'s Meaningful Measures initiative?
    a. Promotion of patient involvement in care planning
    b. Elimination of racial bias in program planning
    c. Attention to issues with potential for improvement
    d. Improvement of data systems

25. How does the Pareto principle relate to outcome analyses in a healthcare institution?
    a. It is predicted that 80 percent of the cost centers will exceed their budgeted total by 20 percent.
    b. The areas with the largest number of employees tend to have the greatest variations in performance measures.
    c. Up to 80 percent of the variations in performance measures are due to only 20 percent of areas that are measured.
    d. The areas with the largest number of employees tend to have the smallest variations in performance measures.

26. Which of the following should alert nursing staff to the possibility of an infant abduction attempt?
    a. A nurse is carrying the infant in the hallway.
    b. The mother has removed the blanket with the security tag.
    c. The CMA says that the infant's name bracelet came off during a diaper change.
    d. The father forgot his name badge.

27. The hospital would be penalized for the 30-day readmission of which of the following diagnoses?
    a. Abdominal surgery for colon cancer
    b. Right total knee arthroplasty
    c. Sepsis due to multiple trauma
    d. End-stage renal disease

28. The AHRQ (Agency for Healthcare Research and Quality) has published quality standards that define the safety culture of a healthcare system. Which of the following standards is viewed as the most controversial?
    a. Strive for safety in an admittedly high-risk environment.
    b. Involve individuals at all levels of the agency hierarchy.
    c. Commit sufficient resources to achieve safety goals.
    d. Maintain a blame-free framework for error reporting.

29. A manager is addressing the Lean criteria for performance improvement. Which of the following strategies would address the People mode?
    a. Requiring managers to communicate process change requirements to all employees
    b. Including employees in the process evaluation decisions
    c. Contracting with the vendor with the lowest price
    d. Limiting stakeholders' evaluation of process changes

30. Which of the following choices is consistent with the Medicaid regulations for provider-preventable conditions (PPCs) and other provider-preventable conditions (OPPCs)?
    a. Hospital care-acquired conditions (HCACs) such as pressure ulcers are designated as OPPCs.
    b. PPCs relate to inpatient care, and OPPCs relate to either inpatient or outpatient care.
    c. Surgical site infection following joint replacement is considered an OPPC.
    d. Reimbursement schedules for PPCs and OPPCs are set by the individual states.

31. Which of the following choices identifies the most critical outcome of patient-care documentation?
    a. Use of the EHR makes it easier for nursing supervisors to monitor staff compliance.
    b. Utilization of specialized equipment is documented.
    c. Supply levels depend on documentation of usage for adequate replacement.
    d. Value-based reimbursement plans depend on accurate documentation.

32. A just culture model has been proposed to address the inequities of the blame-free approach to error reporting. Which of the following behaviors is addressed in this model?
    a. Forgetting a step
    b. Omitting a step
    c. Disregarding the protocol
    d. All of the above

33. The team is identifying goals to address the improvement of a specific process. Which of the following goals is stated correctly?
    a. Hospital readmission rates will decrease over the next quarter.
    b. CAUTI infections will be zero for the second quarter.
    c. Patient reports of adequate pain control will increase 10 percent in the next quarter.
    d. Community feedback will be positive.

34. Which of the following choices would be an appropriate outcome for an organizational safety goal aimed at harm reduction?
    a. Improved access to healthcare information
    b. Empowerment of the workforce
    c. Reduction of duplicate services
    d. Improved rate of medication errors

35. The project team is planning the implementation of the patient-portal online access for a healthcare system. The team will use a Gantt chart to organize the project. What is the first step in the development of this chart?
    a. Identify all managers with responsibility for the project.
    b. Acquire all materials required for each level of the project.
    c. Construct outcome measures for each stage of the project.
    d. Create a work-breakdown structure.

36. Which of the following data management systems consolidates patient-care information from multiple sources?
    a. Healthcare Customer Relations Management (HCRM) system
    b. Enterprise Application software
    c. Electronic Health Record (EHR)
    d. Reliability Centered Management system

37. Which of the following safety interventions has demonstrated the <u>least</u> positive effect on error rates?
    a. SBAR communication
    b. Greater resources for training
    c. Safety teams in individual nursing units
    d. Senior management unit visits

38. The acronyms PDCA (Plan, Do, Check, Act) and PDSA (Plan, Do, Study, Act) are often used interchangeably. How is the PDSA model different than the PDCA model?
    a. The PDSA model is used more effectively in human services industries.
    b. The PDSA model was originally designed as a continuous improvement model.
    c. The PDSA model provides more reliable estimates of project outcomes.
    d. The PDSA model compares results to expected outcomes.

39. What is the main function of program champions?
    a. Management of cost-reduction initiatives
    b. Maintenance of stakeholder relationships
    c. Management of nursing staff contract negotiations
    d. Monitoring of root cause analysis for fall injuries

40. What is the most basic requirement for any data management system?
    a. Standardized data collection methods
    b. Elimination of human error in data entry
    c. Use of the system that competitors are using
    d. Estimation of CMS incentive payments

41. According to the American Hospital Association's Triple Aim, what is the intended outcome of an alliance among an acute-care hospital system, primary care providers, and specialty providers?
    a. Shared financial risk to reduce the per capita costs
    b. Decreased emergency room visits
    c. Improved revenue stream for all participants
    d. Improved employee retention

42. In the Six Sigma process improvement model, the role of process champion also may be used to label which of the following team roles?
    a. Facilitator
    b. Sponsor
    c. Team Leader
    d. Scribe

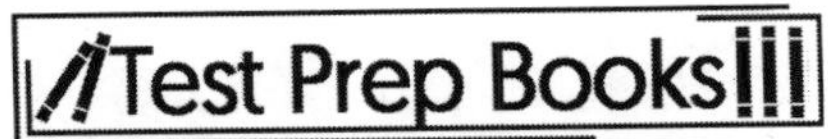

43. A large healthcare system in the Northeast was recently fined more than eighteen million dollars for a HIPPA violation related to the security of the system websites. Which of the following choices is consistent with that error?

a. Data sharing between providers was blocked.
b. Patient data was accessible to third parties.
c. Excessive time elapsed between testing and posting of results.
d. Inaccurate data was not corrected in a timely manner.

44. Which of the following elements is MOST critical to effective organizational priority setting?

a. Stakeholder interests
b. Objectives
c. Timing
d. Resources

45. Who is responsible for the development of a hospital's emergency preparedness plans?

a. The Centers for Medicare & Medicaid Services (CMS)
b. The Centers for Disease Control and Prevention (CDC)
c. The American Hospital Association (AHA)
d. The individual hospital

46. Intravenous infusion pumps are programmed to deliver a set volume of solution each hour. The pump's alarm signals when the infusion is complete, when the solution meets any resistance due to infiltration of the solution into the tissue, and when the battery is expired. Which of the following incidents is most commonly associated with pump failure?

a. Unauthorized user
b. Alarm fatigue
c. Battery explosion
d. Unclear interface

47. Which of the following statements is consistent with the development of an organizational action plan?

a. There needs to be a separate action plan for each major element of the organizational structure.
b. Development of employee action plans is focused on contractual issues rather than project planning.
c. In large organizations, the action plan is only used to identify those responsible for each element of the plan.
d. Action plans for individual groups in an organization are considered stand-alone plans that address specific problems for that group.

48. Which of the following choices is consistent with the project charter for a quality improvement program?

a. It is an outline of the entire quality improvement plan.
b. The document is legally binding.
c. It requires unique performance measures.
d. It is developed by and for senior managers.

49. Which of the following choices is consistent with the purpose of the 2016 National Strategy for Healthcare initiative?
    a. Improve end-of-life care
    b. Promote lifelong learning for all providers
    c. Promote active participation of patients and families
    d. Improve IT infrastructure

50. The acronym CIA—confidentiality, integrity, and accessibility—refers to the priorities of information security in a healthcare institution. Which of the following choices is an example of a breach of confidentiality?
    a. Data entry errors in the EHR
    b. Restricted interdepartmental data sharing
    c. Unsecured mobile nursing computers
    d. Complicated app and device syncing

51. Which of the following choices is an example of a balancing measure as used in a quality improvement project?
    a. Number of defective items per 1000 pieces delivered last quarter
    b. Percentage of orders completed on deadline
    c. Customer satisfaction rating for a new product
    d. Comparison of actual cost to estimated cost per unit

52. Which of the following statements is consistent with the process of credentialing?
    a. The leadership team evaluates the clinical performance of all licensed providers.
    b. State boards determine the scope of practice for licensed providers.
    c. Credentialing requires that all providers must be licensed and certified in their specialty.
    d. All applicants who are properly licensed must be accepted by the leadership team.

53. Leaders are assessing the KPIs for a newly opened trauma unit. The average patient stay in the trauma unit is 48 hours greater than in the clinical pathway model. Which of the following choices is a potential special cause variation for this example?
    a. The Level 1 trauma center's transfer policy
    b. The RN staffing levels on all shifts
    c. The availability of surgical suites
    d. An average patient age range of twenty-five to seventy-six

54. All personnel wear name tags. What additional safety strategies can be used to increase the efficiency of the staff identification methods?
    a. Color-coding is changed according to a random schedule
    b. Embedded door codes are randomly reassigned
    c. Require agency-provided scrubs
    d. All of the above

55. The group is developing an action plan for improving compliance with eye health guidelines for patients with diabetes. Which of the following choices would be an appropriate indicator for this plan?
    a. Patients with diabetes will have decreased progression of retinopathy.
    b. The patient compliance with twice-yearly eye checks will improve.
    c. Reminder messages will be sent to all patients with diabetes.
    d. The number of ophthalmology visits will be tracked in the patient portals.

56. What is the principal market condition that has prompted the expansion of the scope of the risk management process for healthcare organizations?
    a. Value-based care models
    b. Diagnosis-related groups (DRGs)
    c. Fee-for-service services
    d. Escalating legal costs

57. Which of the following activities would be appropriate to introduce a QI initiative?
    a. Implement the change based on an executive consensus.
    b. Broadcast an email message to announce policy changes.
    c. Add the new performance criteria to the employee handbook.
    d. Conduct an information session for interested employees.

58. Which of the following choices is NOT an intended function of the Control Chart?
    a. Identify areas for possible improvement.
    b. Conduct root cause analysis of process failure.
    c. Evaluate the effectiveness of new initiatives.
    d. Monitor sustainability of improved processes.

59. Which of the following statements is consistent with the structure and/or function of the Academy of Healthcare Research and Quality (AHRQ)?
    a. The agency has statutory power to enforce practice guidelines.
    b. The agency is funded by private sector donors.
    c. The agency provides toolkits for quality improvement.
    d. The agency's database use is restricted to funded researchers.

60. The government has published a risk assessment tool (SRA) to be used for agency risk assessment efforts. Which of the following choices is INCORRECT?
    a. The assessment is required by the HIPAA Security Rule.
    b. This instrument is best for larger systems.
    c. The SRA identifies potential areas of risk.
    d. The data is used to devise a mitigation plan.

61. There has been criticism of the Six Sigma approach to performance improvement. Which of the following issues is modifiable?
    a. The protocol is expensive in terms of time and resources.
    b. The initiatives often fail.
    c. The program is difficult to learn.
    d. Customer satisfaction is difficult to predict.

62. Healthcare managers have adopted the fishbone diagram from the Toyota business model that provides a framework for root cause analysis. Which of the following choices is consistent with this diagram?
    a. Team members must be quality improvement experts.
    b. Human error is always identified as one of the “causes” by the model.
    c. The analysis is commonly used for staff evaluation and punitive action.
    d. The success of the model depends on an accurate problem statement.

63. Which of the following describes the Science of Improvement as defined by the Institute for Healthcare Improvement (IHI)?
    a. The improvement process is focused on root cause error analysis.
    b. The process uses the plan, do, study, act (PDSA) sequence to identify areas of improvement.
    c. The successful implementation of the improvement plan can be tied to CMS reimbursement.
    d. The process is more appropriate for inpatient care settings than primary care settings.

64. Pareto analysis can generate a prioritized action plan. Which dimension of other action plans is NOT part of the Pareto analysis?
    a. Estimation of costs associated with the implementation of the plan
    b. Identification of interested stakeholders and employees
    c. Prioritization of the problem list
    d. Comparison of group performance

65. Which of the following choices is consistent with the characteristics of a high-reliability healthcare organization?
    a. The organization has no reported system failures for extended periods.
    b. Work processes are reduced to the simplest form possible.
    c. Senior management is responsible for risk assessment and quality improvement.
    d. Success is measured in terms of near-misses.

66. Which of the following is consistent with the mission of the National Quality Forum (NQF)?
    a. The forum is funded by the United States government.
    b. The NQF develops communication plans aimed at improved safety.
    c. Only specialty providers can approve the use of new NQF measures.
    d. NQF measures are used to evaluate patient care in multiple settings.

67. The group is conducting a root cause analysis of a discrepancy in the reporting of the controlled substance counts on a specific nursing unit. Which of the following choices would be an organizational cause for this error?
    a. The count was signed by a single RN instead of two licensed personnel.
    b. The count could not be completed because the computers were down.
    c. There was no agency protocol for controlled substance reconciliation.
    d. The RN signed for a dose that wasn't used or discarded.

68. Which of the following choices is consistent with risk-adjustment methods?
    a. They were developed to accommodate the Affordable Care Act.
    b. They are only used to adjust the effect of age on outcome measures.
    c. They project costs based on factors beyond the provider’s control.
    d. They are used only by third-party payers.

69. A group facilitator is concerned that the current action plan does not reflect the customer's viewpoint. Which of the following measures is specifically designed to provide this information?

a. Cause and effect analysis
b. CATWOE analysis
c. Risk Analysis
d. Impact Analysis

70. What is the role of the World Health Organization (WHO) concerning safe care?

a. The WHO stresses the need for the application of research results to improve health.
b. The WHO issues pandemic regulations that require one hundred percent compliance by member nations.
c. The WHO case manages all active TB infections.
d. The WHO conducts vaccine development for newly identified infections.

71. A provider wants to develop a visual representation of the ages of diabetic patients and the number of clinic visits in the past year. Which of the following tools could display that information?

a. Scatter diagram
b. Fishbone diagram
c. Control chart
d. Pareto chart

72. What is the definition of a process control?

a. Any assessment measure that avoids errors at the customer level
b. A measure that identifies links among specific causes
c. A process that evaluates employee performance outcomes
d. A time and motion study of the new manufacturing procedure

73. What is the most significant risk associated with canceled patient appointments that are not rescheduled?

a. Lost agency revenue
b. Staffing issues
c. Patient outcomes
d. CMS evaluation

74. Which of the following choices is consistent with the Healthcare Effectiveness Data and Information Set (HEDIS) databases that are developed by the National Committee for Quality Assurance (NCQA)?

a. HEDIS data tracks the incidence of communicable diseases in a population.
b. HEDIS measures hospital compliance with environmental standards.
c. HEDIS data is used to evaluate the effectiveness of healthcare plans.
d. HEDIS data does not currently track Electronic Health Record (EHR) usage in Special Needs Plans (SNPs).

75. Process champions must be skilled in many different areas of organizational management. When assessing the performance of a process champion in a healthcare system, which of the following qualities may be difficult to measure objectively?
   a. Establishing the patient connection
   b. Mentoring new team members
   c. Maintaining the connection between team members and senior management
   d. Separating personal vision from institutional priorities

76. What is the key element (or elements) that distinguishes enterprise risk management (ERM) from earlier healthcare risk management models?
   a. Cybersecurity is now included in the risk assessment.
   b. Patient outcomes are the driving force.
   c. Strategic planning assessment is included.
   d. All of the above are correct.

77. The team leaders of the 20/20 Eye Care center are discussing marketing strategies. Which of the following choices is a structural measure associated with this process?
   a. Percentage of patients over forty-five who were screened for glaucoma
   b. Number of full-time and part-time board-certified providers
   c. Hospital admissions from the ambulatory surgical center
   d. Annual rate of post-operative infections

78. Which of the following statements is consistent with the effect of change theory on quality improvement?
   a. When the purpose of a proposed quality innovation is well articulated, diffusion is rapid.
   b. **Early adopters** of quality improvement innovations are often group leaders.
   c. **Late majority** adopters quickly recognize the potential of the proposed changes.
   d. **Diffusion** cannot occur without prior formal **dissemination** of information.

79. Which of the following choices is a business value-added activity?
   a. Accommodating government-mandated safety requirements
   b. Completing client-specific product configurations
   c. Updating risk management protocols
   d. Revising a defective prototype

80. The I-PASS mnemonic was developed to improve quality of communication in the patient handoff, which has been identified as an area of significant risk. According to the model, which of the following handoff statements is consistent with "situation awareness"?
   a. "The patient is scheduled for a CT of the head at 9 AM."
   b. "The patient is stable and was admitted with an upper GI bleed yesterday."
   c. "The patient is a 59-year-old male with acute MI, stable vital signs, no pain, and is resting."
   d. "Based on my assessment, he needs a chest x-ray to check for pneumonia today."

81. Which of the following patients would qualify for the disease management model of case management?
   a. A 75-year-old female patient with right knee arthroplasty
   b. A 62-year-old male patient with a right-sided hemorrhagic stroke
   c. A 49-year-old male patient with a posterior wall myocardial infarction
   d. A 45-year-old female patient with tumor lysis syndrome

82. Which of the following choices is consistent with the Pareto chart?
   a. The chart is used to identify common cause and special cause variation.
   b. The chart can only be used effectively in the problem identification phase of quality improvement.
   c. The Pareto chart requires interval-level variables.
   d. The results of the Pareto chart identify areas for improvement.

83. Which of the following choices is a common cause variation according to SPC (statistical process control) measurement?
   a. Environmental variations
   b. Human error
   c. Machine malfunctions
   d. Variations in materials

84. Communication errors in patient hand-off situations are estimated to be the root cause for as many as seventy-five percent of all sentinel events. Using the IPASS reporting format, if a patient were experiencing chest pain, where would that information be reported?
   a. I
   b. P
   c. A
   d. S

85. The end product of the 5 Whys technique is the identification of a countermeasure. How is a countermeasure different than a solution?
   a. Countermeasures assess blame.
   b. Countermeasures address the root cause.
   c. Countermeasures are less difficult to implement.
   d. Countermeasures must be evaluated by managers.

86. According to the I-PASS model, which of the following choices is consistent with "illness severity"?
   a. The 79-year-old male is being treated with warfarin for A-fib, and he is a watcher.
   b. The patient is scheduled for a CT scan today.
   c. The patient will need skilled nurses' visits when discharged.
   d. The patient will need new IV orders if the infusion is to be continued.

87. Which of the following is consistent with the purpose of registries for healthcare data management?
   a. Allowing data sharing among multiple healthcare systems
   b. Collecting data about specific patient conditions for quality care innovation
   c. Capturing care costs for reimbursement
   d. Tracking of provider reimbursement schedules

88. What is the primary focus of the CMS Meaningful Measures 2022 initiative?
    a. Identification of potential areas for quality improvement
    b. Fee schedules for patients covered by CMS services
    c. Primary care preventive medicine best practices
    d. Surgical readmission rates

89. Scorecards and dashboards are used to measure organizational effectiveness. Which of the following choices is consistent with these reports?
    a. Scorecards can identify root cause.
    b. Dashboards address structural outcomes.
    c. Both measures provide actionable data.
    d. Both measures have "drill-down" capability.

90. The team leader is tracking the number of conversions for several social media websites. Which of the following choices is the best engagement metric for that question?
    a. Likes
    b. Follows
    c. Direct messages
    d. Social shares

91. Concerning HIPAA reporting, which technical safeguards address access to protected health information (PHI)?
    a. Integrity controls
    b. Audit controls
    c. Transmission security
    d. All of the above

92. Which of the following would be tracked on a scorecard?
    a. Telemetry unit census
    b. Current ER wait time
    c. 30-day readmissions
    d. L&D nurse-to-patient ratio

93. The IHI identified six patient-care qualities to serve as benchmarks for addressing healthcare disparities. Which of the following is NOT included in that list?
    a. Timeliness
    b. Effectiveness
    c. Efficiency
    d. Cost control

94. ISO 9000 (International Organization for Standardization) is a non-governmental agency that publishes standards for more than one thousand goods and services. This list also includes the principles of quality management. Which of the following is NOT one of the characteristics of this model?
    a. Relationships with employees
    b. Product quality
    c. Customer-first attitude
    d. Organizational QI mindset

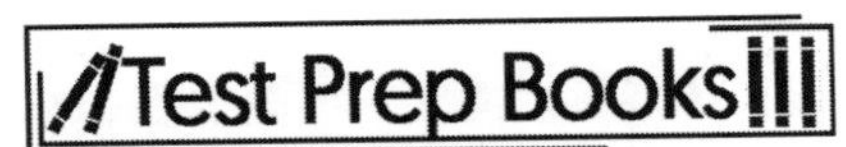

95. Which of the following statements about sampling is correct?
   a. Probability samples are more prone to bias.
   b. Convenience sampling is a non-probability sampling method.
   c. Voluntary sampling is a form of probability sampling.
   d. Random data is required for non-probability sampling.

96. Electronic Clinical Quality Measures (eCQMs) include abstracted data from the hospital's EHR system that are submitted to CMS to demonstrate patient-care effectiveness. These measures are submitted in addition to mandatory quality measures, and the hospital can voluntarily decide which eCQMs to report. Which of the following choices is an example of a voluntary eCQM?
   a. Infants who are bottle-fed exclusively from birth to discharge
   b. ICU patients who are diagnosed with new pressure ulcers
   c. Time in minutes from ER admission decision to patient transfer to the nursing unit
   d. Patients who are discharged with one or more new opioid medications

97. When comparing Lean with Six Sigma, which one of the following statements is consistent with Lean?
   a. Lean philosophy is focused on waste control.
   b. Lean uses more advanced analytic procedures.
   c. Lean assesses data for variation or outliers.
   d. Lean is best employed after Six Sigma analysis.

98. Which of the following is consistent with the hospital's use of outside sources for data analysis?
   a. Outside performance data may be biased.
   b. Generating the data in-house is less expensive.
   c. Creating tables helps to identify importing errors.
   d. Formatting issues affect data quality.

99. What is the purpose of the Employee Net Promoter Scale (eNPS)?
   a. To assess employee compliance with required continuing education requirements
   b. To quantify employee use of the Human Resources information portal
   c. To identify employees that are dissatisfied with their job
   d. To evaluate employee use of the internet during regular business hours

100. Which of the following statements regarding the current state of cybersecurity in many healthcare systems is consistent with industry cyber security expert assessments?
   a. HIPAA technical standards are insufficient for the current threat level.
   b. Access controls are adequate to the threat.
   c. EHR platforms from leading vendors are secure.
   d. Two-factor authorization is not required for associate partners of the system.

101. Which of the following statements is true about benchmarking?
   a. All stakeholders are included in the evaluation process.
   b. All benchmarks are chosen by senior managers.
   c. JCAHO sets all agency benchmarks.
   d. Benchmarking only applies to acute-care facilities.

102. Which of the following Health Insurance Portability and Accountability Act of 1996 (HIPAA) violations could result in a ten-year prison sentence?

a. Hospital clerical staff sells social security numbers.
b. Hospital staff accesses the EHR record of a “celebrity” patient.
c. A newly hired nursing assistant takes home worksheets with identifiable patient information.
d. Patient pages are left open on the computer when the nurse is called to an emergency in the next room.

103. The team is using the SWOT (Strengths, Weaknesses, Opportunities, and Threats) model to consider adding additional services to their product line. Which of the following choices would be considered an "external - helpful" factor?

a. Existing organizational resources
b. Knowledge gained from past failures
c. Federal pandemic relief funds
d. Loss of customers due to supply chain issues

104. The PETT instrument (people, environment, tools, task) is used in human systems engineering to identify the entire scope of a process, including the interactions among patients, staff, and families. The model also identifies facilitators and barriers to successful outcomes. Which of the following barriers is an environmental issue?

a. Language barrier
b. Insufficient staff
c. Complex device instructions
d. Departmental conflicts

105. Which of the following choices would not satisfy provider compliance with any of the Meaningful Use criteria?

a. E-prescribing of medications
b. Reimbursement schedules
c. Interagency EHR connectivity
d. A1C results for diabetic patients

106. Which of the following choices is NOT one of the most common “ribs” of the fishbone diagram?

a. Materials
b. Methods
c. Costs
d. Environment

107. Which of the following principles is associated with the Agile project management protocol?

a. The product is delivered in its final form.
b. Customer-generated alterations are discouraged.
c. The most common marketing strategy is through social media.
d. Positive outcomes depend on daily interaction with customers.

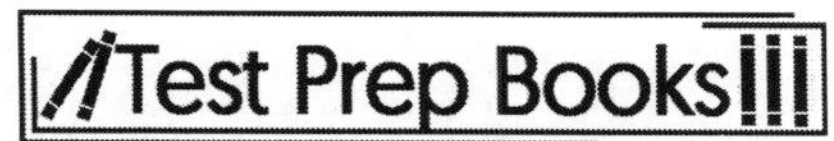

108. Which of the following issues related to the interstate regulation of telemedicine is state-specific?
   a. Technology availability
   b. Software licensing
   c. Medicare payments
   d. Licensing restrictions for MDs and RNs

109. Which of the following organizational culture types is most common in successful start-up companies?
   a. Clan culture
   b. Adhocracy
   c. Hierarchy
   d. Market

110. What is the most significant advantage of multi-stage sampling for data management?
   a. Large groups are sampled more efficiently.
   b. It works best with homogenous populations.
   c. The method eliminates population bias.
   d. The method requires a pre-determined sample size.

111. Which of the following choices is consistent with Kotter's Change Theory?
   a. Creating a vision and strategy for change requires first removing the obstacles.
   b. The members of the coalition should be senior managers.
   c. Rewarding small behavioral changes leads to greater success.
   d. Communicating the vision is the final step of the process.

112. In a company with a hierarchical culture, the employees would be involved in which of the following steps of organizational planning?
   a. Contingency planning
   b. Operational planning
   c. Tactical planning
   d. Strategic Planning

113. What is the purpose of the Hospital Readmissions Reduction Program (HRRP)?
   a. To track thirty-day readmission rates of all patients covered by Medicaid
   b. To estimate costs for patients with end-stage renal disease
   c. To encourage hospitals to improve communication
   d. To provide patient-education models for chronic disease

114. Which of the following choices is consistent with the concept of resiliency in high-reliability healthcare systems?
   a. Respect for individual work product
   b. Effective mitigation strategies
   c. Prompt feedback for all employee concerns
   d. Comprehensive educational resources

115. Which of the following functions is the most common reason for using a virtual private network (VPN) in place of a conventional network?
   a. It is a private email network for senior managers.
   b. The system accommodates remote staff positions.
   c. It protects against unauthorized system access.
   d. It is used to stream patient teaching modules.

116. Which of the following choices is consistent with the Physician Value-Based Modifier (PVBM) program?
   a. Provider groups accept all financial risk.
   b. Providers are reimbursed for the quality rather than the number of patient-care encounters.
   c. Hospitals are rewarded for timely discharge of preterm infants covered by Medicaid.
   d. Hospitals can opt out of the program.

117. The team decides to create a process map to monitor the progress of a project. The team is particularly interested in tracking the availability of all necessary resources and the identification of waste that may be occurring at any point in the process. Which of the following process maps is the best choice for the team?
   a. Value stream map
   b. Basic flow chart
   c. Value chain map
   d. Cross functional map

118. Value-based care models are associated with varying degrees of financial risk. Which of the following choices is consistent with the definitions of upside risk and downside risk?
   a. Upside risk is associated with penalties for failure to meet metrics.
   b. CMS can limit participation in downside risk models.
   c. Plans that assume downside risk must be well coordinated to be successful.
   d. Downside risk models are not penalized for failure to meet CMS benchmarks.

119. Which of the following choices explains how stratified sampling decreases variability?
   a. Simple random selection
   b. Homogenous strata
   c. Self-enrolled strata
   d. Restricted sample size

120. Which of the following choices is consistent with BPM (Business Process Management)?
   a. BPM is an informal annual review of all customer satisfaction data for senior managers.
   b. The Business Process Champion is responsible for only a retrospective review of processes.
   c. Six Sigma expertise for team members is not required or encouraged.
   d. The continuous review process assumes that people store plans in their heads.

121. Which of the following choices is consistent with the use of control charts?
   a. The chart tracks structural measures.
   b. Stable processes are not tracked.
   c. Special cause variations cannot be identified
   d. Control charts identify areas for improvement.

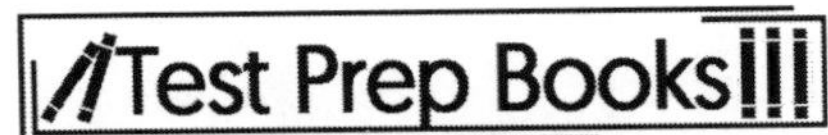

122. Which of the following choices identifies the CMS benchmark for the transition of care from the hospital to the home environment?
   a. Preventing early readmission
   b. Verifying the medication list
   c. Self-regulating chronic diseases
   d. Providing timely follow-up care

123. A team is using the VMOSA framework (Vision, Mission, Objectives, Strategies, and Action Plans) to develop an organizational action plan for a company that sells widgets. Which of the following choices is a mission statement?
   a. The company will market products that increase leisure time for the entire family.
   b. The company will provide quality products that meet customers' expectations through continuous process improvement.
   c. There will be a thirty percent increase in customer satisfaction at the end of the next quarter.
   d. The team will use the eighty-twenty rule to focus the action plan.

124. Which data management system could be used to track OSHA compliance?
   a. Reliability Centered Maintenance (RCM) system
   b. Enterprise Application Software
   c. Electronic Healthcare Record (EHR)
   d. Healthcare Customer Relations Management (HCRM) software

125. Healthcare economists predict that Medicare costs will continue to increase because existing care plans do not successfully integrate social services. Which of the following choices is suggested as a solution to this deficiency?
   a. Increasing Medicare payments for using social determinants of health as benchmarks
   b. Using EHR data to identify individual patient needs
   c. Mandatory reporting of patients' employment and housing status
   d. Actively enrolling all Medicaid patients in qualifying programs

# Answer Explanations #2

**1. C:** Institutional quality is measured by key performance indicators (KPIs), which means that any effort aimed at improving or maintaining quality must be tied to a specific KPI. The strategy phase of the strategic quality planning process identifies all of the project's specific steps, and the research phase includes the analysis of the data that forms the basis for the project. This means that Choices *A* and *B* are incorrect. Choice *D* is incorrect because the strategic quality planning process has two phases: the research phase and the strategy phase.

**2. C:** Effective data analysis requires the preparation of the raw data. One of the preparatory steps is the data cleansing process, which includes the correction of readily apparent documentation errors. Data exploration includes searching individual databases for unanticipated findings, which means that Choice *A* is incorrect. Data blending is the process of merging datasets to identify novel information that results from the combined sources. This means that Choice *B* is incorrect. Data aggregation from multiple sources follows an extract, transfer, and load sequence. Therefore, Choice *D* is incorrect.

**3. B:** Activities that are both urgent and important are commonly associated with a specific deadline or element of time. That means that stepping in to moderate a panel discussion in place of a colleague who is suddenly taken ill would be important because there are possible consequences if the discussion were not moderated, and it would be urgent because of the immediacy of the event. Choice *A* is incorrect because although the project is important, there is no immediate need to complete the planning of the project. Choice *C* is incorrect because the Instagram invitation may or may not be important, and it does not require an immediate response. Choice *D* is neither urgent nor important because according to the model, the time could be better spent answering and sending messages.

**4. B:** Mechanistic organizations take a rigid approach to problem-solving that often results in a less effective response to the changing organizational demands and employees who are not encouraged to reach their potential. This rigid approach is the result of centralized leadership that depends on rigid protocols and top-down communication, which serves to discourage or eliminate employee involvement in planning and problem-solving. The remaining choices describe leadership styles that depend on empowering each individual in the organization. Values-based leadership involves supporting individual equality and liberty that can result in social change, which means that Choice *A* is incorrect. Choice *C* is incorrect because organic organizations, which are viewed as the opposite of mechanistic organizations, depend on lateral communication to encourage input from individual employees. As noted, values-based leadership and transformational leadership encourage the active participation of the individual employee, which is common to the organic organization rather than the mechanistic organization; therefore, Choice *D* is incorrect.

**5. A:** The facilitator assigns portions of the agenda to individuals with the appropriate expertise to expedite the discussion. The alternate speaker presents the content and answers questions from the group. This strategy also encourages group participation. While team members do gain experience, the intended outcome for this strategy is to provide expert content expeditiously; therefore, Choice *B* is incorrect. The facilitator needs to be knowledgeable about the content, choose the right person to present the information, and clear all scheduling constraints. This means that Choice *C* is incorrect because delegating this portion of the agenda potentially adds work for the facilitator. Although the facilitator should strive to maintain the attention of the group, the purpose of delegating a portion of the agenda is to improve time management; therefore, Choice *D* is incorrect.

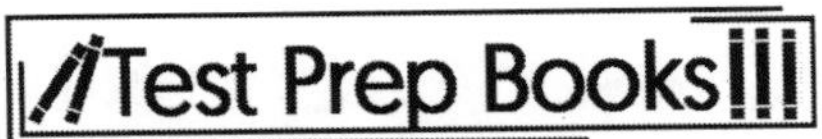

**6. D:** The NQF developed the e-measures to transition data analysis results from paper and pencil to electronic reporting. The NQF published 113 measures; however, a guide for developing new e-measures (the Measure Authoring Tool, or MAT) was also published for IT team leaders. This authoring tool guides the development of additional tools by measurement specialists. The NQF reviews the e-measures and posts updates every three years, but it does not monitor the usage of the e-measures, which means that Choice *A* is incorrect. Hospitals are free to use the MAT to develop hospital-specific e-measures, which means that Choice *B* is incorrect. CMS originally adopted 44 of the available measures, which means that Choice *C* is incorrect.

**7. D:** Benchmarking is the process of assessing the strategic planning activities of a competing organization. This information is used to weigh different options rather than as a planning blueprint. Choice *A* is incorrect because the voice of the customer is a separate form of evaluation that differs from benchmarking. The voice of the customer is measured in satisfaction surveys or other face-to-face situations, and the resulting information impacts the quality planning process in a different way than benchmarking. Because no two organizations are identical, the information acquired through benchmarking is viewed only as a general view of what was successful or unsuccessful for a similar organization. This means that Choice *B* is incorrect. Price controls would not be identified in the benchmarking process, which means that Choice *C* is incorrect.

**8. C**: The affinity diagram would be a useful first step for this meeting because the diagram identifies common themes among the solutions that provide a starting point for the multi-voting process; therefore, Choice *C* is the correct answer. The Eisenhower matrix is used by the individual to prioritize tasks and would not be useful in the stated scenario, so Choice *A* is incorrect. Multivoting provides individuals the ability to make personal decisions about the identified solutions as part of the larger group. Small group discussion would limit the possible decisions about any single issue; therefore, Choice *B* is incorrect. Brainstorming sessions are often used before multivoting to identify the possible solutions or ideas that are to be addressed in the multivoting process, so Choice *D* is incorrect.

**9. C:** The success of the IHI data collection plan depends on the collection of accurate data; however, the collection plan is not based on a stringent research protocol. Choice *A* is incorrect because the use of existing data for the analysis is strongly recommended since collecting new data requires additional time and money. Sampling saves time and resources, and the sample size is an estimate of the population rather than a mathematical calculation. Therefore, Choice *B* is incorrect. Team leaders are cautioned to consider the cost-benefit of the analysis; however, the IHI plan is identified as a simple plan that can identify areas for improvement without significant resource investment. This means that Choice *D* is incorrect.

**10. A:** Choice *A* is correct because the AHRQ assessment of a healthcare agency's safety culture addresses many aspects of the delivery of patient care; however, the financial costs are not directly assessed. The survey does assess the opinions of the personnel as well as the safe practices of environmental services and the information technology department, which means that Choices *B* and *C* are incorrect. Choice *D* is incorrect because the rate of temporary staffing is closely related to patient safety, and the issue is addressed in the survey.

**11. A:** Strategic planners are responsible for planning for the current and future needs of the organization. In healthcare, this means that long-term goals can become quickly outdated in the rapidly changing environment, so well-defined short-term goals can be more reliable in measuring the quality of care. Choice *B* is incorrect because the planners are also responsible for including goals set for the organization by other authorities such as the Centers for Medicare and Medicaid Services (CMS). Choice *C* is incorrect because there is no evidence that long-term goals are more successful than short-term goals; however, as noted above, there is evidence that long-term goals often become obsolete. Choice *D* is incorrect because successful healthcare strategists look beyond current circumstances when setting goals and priorities because the future needs most often do not resemble current circumstances.

**12. C:** The facilitator is responsible for providing a plan for follow-through of actions taken. This action should not be delegated to the scribe; therefore, Choice *C* is correct. The remaining activities are consistent with the role of the scribe, which means that Choices *A, B,* and *D* are incorrect.

**13. C:** CMS has set six national goals for healthcare improvement, which are based on four broad principles. Choice *C* is not one of the four broad principles; it is one of the Meaningful Measures established by CMS to improve healthcare delivery while decreasing provider burden. Choices *A, B,* and *D* correctly identify three of the four principles.

**14. B:** Block sampling is the appropriate sampling method for processes that relate to timing or sequencing, and the ER-to-nursing-unit transfer-time policy includes the assessment of both elements. Convenience sampling means that the sample can be chosen from any available source, without regard to the specific sampling requirements for the assessment of transfer times. This means that Choice *A* is incorrect. Self-selection sampling may or may not fulfill the sampling requirement for any inquiry, which means that Choice *C* is incorrect. Systematic sampling is used with large populations for processes that are not sequenced or time-dependent. For example, systematic sampling would be appropriate for assessing documentation of COVID-19 vaccination data for patients over 65 who were admitted in the first quarter. This means that Choice *D* is incorrect.

**15. D:** The key performance indicators (KPIs) are measurable standards that are consistent with the mission and goals of a healthcare organization. These measures vary from one institution to another; however, assessments of financial issues such as bed occupancy rates and patient care issues such as safety are common. Trended data from these assessments can be used to identify areas of weakness in the organization; therefore, Choice *D* is correct. There are performance measures for specific groups in healthcare such as nurses or doctors who practice as primary care providers; however, the institutional KPIs address system-wide issues rather than individual performance. Therefore, Choices *A* and *C* are incorrect. The use of KPIs for performance assessment is not exclusive to large healthcare systems, so Choice *B* is incorrect.

**16. A:** Daily bed turnover rate as compared to national standards is an outcome of the quality of patient care. The remaining choices are incorrect because they are process measures or procedures that meet standards for preventing harm.

**17. A:** CTQs are institutional processes or products that determine customer satisfaction, which is essential to process improvement; therefore, Choice *A* is correct. CMS does not directly affect the identification of the CTQs by the individual institutions, so Choice *B* is incorrect. Institutional profit is assessed through the voice of business (VOB) elements rather than the CTQs; therefore, Choice *C* is incorrect. The research indicates that consideration of both measures is required for optimal process planning, so Choice *D* is incorrect.

**18. A:** Mistake-proofing is the process of identifying specific prevention measures for high-risk patient situations. For instance, the surgical "time out" protocol was developed to prevent surgical errors such

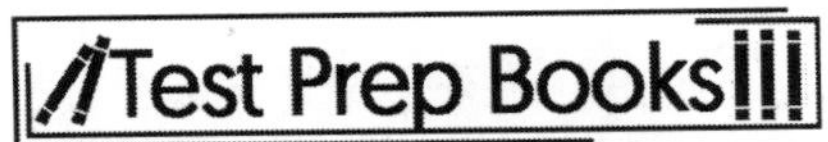

as procedures on the wrong patient, the wrong limb, etc. Mistake-proofing measures consider every possible element of an adverse event to develop a prevention plan. Choice *A* is the correct answer because the "time out" is specific to the prevention of adverse events. Choice *B* is incorrect because the quiet environment rules are aimed at patient satisfaction rather than error prevention. Similarly, Choice *C* is incorrect because the primary purpose for convenient parking options is patient satisfaction rather than error prevention. Scheduling access in a patient portal enhances patient satisfaction and also substantially decreases staffing time spent on scheduling. This means that Choice *D* is incorrect.

**19. C:** The EHR generates Clinical Decision Support (CDS) alerts to the patient's EHR. These alerts include a wide range of information that is relevant to the patient's history and current condition. Based on the patient's data, alerts may be posted to alert the provider that there is an order that may be incorrect or that there is critical documentation that is missing. The importance of these alerts can range from critical to informational; however, there is some indication that many providers ignore the alerts or bypass the system, which means that Choice *C* is correct. Inventory charges are not generally included with the patient-specific data, which means that Choice *A* is incorrect. Choices *B* and *D* are issues for the agency but are not directly related to patient safety and the EHR, so they are incorrect.

**20. B:** Diffusion is the informal transfer of information about a proposed change in policy or process. Team leaders should be alert to the informal transfer of incorrect information. Dissemination is the deliberative process of informing specific groups about the new processes, so Choice *A* is incorrect. Using the new CAUTI bundles is an example of implementation; therefore, Choice *C* is incorrect. Choice *D* is incorrect because spread is defined in terms of the time it takes for a new process to be adopted. Spread can be measured in terms of the rate of compliance.

**21. C:** Stratified sampling requires separating the target population into two homogenous groups and then comparing random samples of each group. Male Medicare patients would be over 65, and annual prostate exams would be an appropriate metric for this relatively homogenous population. Choice *A* is an example of cluster sampling, which uses a random sample of heterogenous population groups. Choice *B* is incorrect because it is an example of systematic sampling, which involves selecting participants from a population according to a recurring interval with a randomly chosen starting point. Volunteer or convenience sampling is a form of non-probability sampling that is subject to bias and does not provide results that can be generalized to the population. This means that Choice *D* is incorrect.

**22. C:** The "time out" is a scripted check of critical details regarding the patient's identity and the intended procedure. It is required a least once before every invasive procedure. The protocol requires that all personnel in the treatment area pause all activity while the checklist is completed by the responsible provider. The "time out" is not to be confused with the consent for a procedure, which is required for all care interventions. This means that Choice *C* is the correct answer. The remaining choices require consent for treatment and two patient identifiers; however, the "time out" is required for procedures that are invasive and associated with possible patient injury. That means that Choices *A*, *B*, and *D* are incorrect.

**23. A:** Central line infection rate is a quantifiable outcome which is the definition of an output. Dressing change modules are activities that are required to meet the proposed objective, so Choice *B* is incorrect. Demonstration of safe practice is an example of an overall objective; therefore, Choice *C* is incorrect. Patient report measures related to pain management are an example of a measurement tool used to evaluate each objective in the action plan, so Choice *D* is incorrect.

**24. C:** The goal of Meaningful Measures is to identify problem areas that have improvement potential. For instance, if the endoscopy department has frequent "no-show" patients, implementing a detailed reminder system could increase patient satisfaction with scheduling and save time and money on staffing. The meaningful measures address organization-specific problem areas that are often related to payment models. Choice *A* is incorrect because the promotion of patient and family involvement in care planning is one of the goals of the CMS National Quality Strategy for Healthcare, rather than the Meaningful Measures initiative. Choices *B* and *D* are incorrect because these measures are general organizing principles for the 2016 CMS National Quality Strategy for Healthcare rather than specific areas for improvement in a single organization.

**25. C:** The Pareto principle states that 80 percent of the variation in performance measures will be due to variations in only 20 percent of the areas that are measured. Application of this principle helps to identify the areas that require improvement; therefore, Choice *C* is correct. In healthcare, the application of the principle is related to variations in performance measures rather than financial details, so Choice *A* is incorrect. The Pareto principle addresses the variation in performance measures not the size of the group; therefore, Choices *B* and *D* are incorrect.

**26: A:** Infants should always be transported in the bassinet for safety reasons and because it indicates that only authorized individuals are caring for the infant. That means that Choice *A* is the correct answer. The nurse educates the family on the importance of all safeguards related to the infant's security. Security tags may be attached to linens and clothing as well as the infant's umbilical clamp. Choice *B* is incorrect because there is no risk to the infant. Choice *C* is incorrect because the CMA reported the incident so that the infant's bracelet could be replaced immediately. Choice *D* is incorrect because the father would need to provide two forms of identification to receive a temporary badge for the duration of his visit. Additionally, infant abduction is most often committed by a stranger.

**27. B:** The HRRP requires reporting of the thirty-day readmission rates for total knee and hip arthroplasty, chronic obstructive lung disease, coronary bypass surgery, acute MI, pneumonia, and heart failure. Financial penalties may be assessed, and hospitals are also required to submit remediation plans for all deficiencies. The value-based program focuses on the need for improved discharge planning to eliminate preventable readmissions. Choices *A, C,* and *D* are incorrect because the readmission rates of the identified diagnoses are not currently tracked by Medicare.

**28. D:** The blame-free environment is critical to safety because, in a punitive environment, the errors that are not reported will be repeated. In light of recent events, nurses have legitimate concerns about the employer approach to error reporting that varies among healthcare systems. This means that Choice *D* is the correct answer. Each of the remaining choices is generally accepted as critical to a culture of safety, which means that they are incorrect.

**29. B:** The People mode addresses relationships with employees, stakeholders, and vendors. Employees from all areas are expected to evaluate work processes and to actively participate in the change process. The Lean principles suggest that the flow of information should not assume a top-down direction because employees at all levels are included in the evaluation of the work processes; therefore, Choice *A* is incorrect. Vendors are also considered to be part of the team, and the quality of the goods and services provided by the vendor would be important considerations in any contractual agreement, so Choice *C* is incorrect. In the Lean model, stakeholders would be involved in the evaluation of proposed process changes, making Choice *D* incorrect.

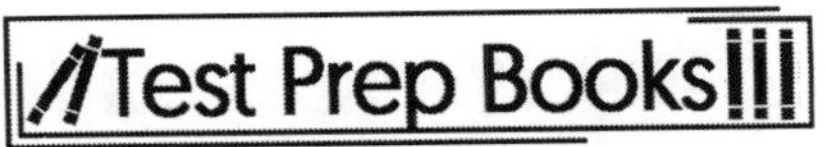

**30. B:** Medicaid designates provider-preventable conditions (PPCs) and other provider-preventable conditions (OPPCs). PPCs include hospital care-acquired conditions (HCACs) such as wound infections and fall injuries. OPPCs occur in either inpatient or outpatient settings and include surgery on the wrong patient, wrong surgery on a patient, and surgery on the wrong limb. Choice *A* is incorrect because HCACs are inpatient injuries that are designated as preventable provider conditions (PPCs). Choice *C* is incorrect because a surgical site infection following joint replacement is an inpatient event that is designated as an HCAC, which does not meet the criteria for the OPPC. Choice *D* is incorrect because increased costs due to PPCs and OPPCs are generally not reimbursed. For instance, if a patient experiences an HCAC such as a wound infection after abdominal surgery, the surgery charges would be reimbursed; however, any additional length of stay or other care costs related to the infection would not be reimbursed. These policies are set by Medicaid and CMS. Individual states can add preventable conditions to the list, but they are prohibited from removing conditions from the list.

**31. D:** Value-based reimbursement schedules are based on analysis of patient-care data. Incomplete or inaccurate documentation affects the bottom line of a hospital. The remaining choices are important documentation functions; however, the critical outcome of adequate documentation is accurate data analysis and reporting of value-based care information. Therefore, Choices *A, B,* and *C* are incorrect.

**32. D:** Modifications to the blame-free approach differentiate between types of errors because there is a difference between unintentional human error, consciously omitting steps, and careless disregard for safe practice. Unsafe practice should be recognized and may require punitive action, depending on the type of error. For instance, nursing practice is regulated by the state nurse practice act, which means that unsafe behaviors such as drug diversion may be punishable by law.

**33. C:** Reliable evaluation results depend on the proper construction of the project goals. Goals should be measurable, specific to the project, achievable, and time-oriented. Choice *C* meets these requirements because it is possible to measure patient reports, and the stated increase in positive reports provides a standard for the evaluation of the goal. Also, while the feasibility of the 10 percent increase will be made by the project team, the increase seems reasonable within the stated time frame. The remaining choices are either incomplete, not achievable or measurable, or not time-oriented. Choice *A* is incorrect because although it is possible that hospital readmission rates could decrease over the next quarter, specifying the rate of improvement would strengthen the evaluation of the goal. Choice *B* is incorrect because zero incidence of catheter-associated urinary tract infections (CAUTI) is not achievable in most in-patient healthcare environments. The final goal is not specific and not measurable as stated, so Choice *D* is incorrect.

**34. D:** Harm reduction refers to adverse events that occur in the actual patient-care environment. The reduction of medication administration errors is an appropriate outcome because it is measurable. The remaining choices are incorrect because the outcomes stated are at the organizational level rather than at the direct patient-care level where harm occurs.

**35. D:** The Gantt chart tracks each element of a project. The first step is the identification of the work breakdown chart that typically includes all of the information identified in Choices *A, B,* and *C*; however, the work breakdown chart is based on the 100 percent rule, which requires the identification of the entire scope of the project from start to completion. Therefore, Choice *D* is correct.

**36. A:** Healthcare Customer Relations Management (HCRM) system software collects and analyzes multiple forms of patient and population data from sources such as the EHR, social media, and consumer sites. This integration provides team leaders with information that can be used in marketing as well as patient care. Enterprise Application software focuses on the needs of the entire hospital system as opposed to the care of the individual patient, so Choice *B* is incorrect. The EHR is a single source that collects and stores in-hospital care documentation. The EHR does not integrate information from consumer sites, which means that Choice *C* is incorrect. Reliability Centered Maintenance software assesses system-wide equipment performance. For instance, the software can estimate equipment maintenance schedules for the heating system and the risks and possible outcomes of equipment failure. The software does assess patient care, which means that Choice *D* is incorrect.

**37. A:** Communication defects are responsible for a disproportionate amount of error in the healthcare setting. The SBAR framework (situation, background, assessment, recommendation) was developed by physicians to standardize reporting from one individual to another. Recent research suggests that the model may improve communication, but any positive effect on errors in the clinical setting is lacking. The model has not had a significant positive effect on errors, so Choice *A* is correct. The remaining choices have demonstrated positive effects on the safety culture; however, the interventions are synergistic, which means that the solution to the problem requires more than one approach to safety. That means that Choices *B, C*, and *D* are incorrect.

**38. C:** The PDCA model was introduced in 1950 by Dr. W Edwards Deming as a way to impose the rigor of scientific inquiry upon business practices. The original intent of the PDCA model was continuous quality improvement. Over time, however, Deming and others proposed the PDSA model because the *Study* phase was more effective than the original *Check* phase of the PDCA model. Deming felt that there needed to be additional reflection on the results of early testing. This means that Choice *C* is correct because the *Study* phase facilitates more reliable estimates of project outcomes. Choice *A* is incorrect because both models have been used in multiple settings. Of the two models, the PDCA was originally designed as a continuous improvement method, so Choice *B* is incorrect. Choice *D* is incorrect because the PDSA model was specifically designed to go beyond checking and comparing to reflecting on the test results.

**39. B:** A program champion is most often a senior manager who develops and maintains close relationships with existing and potential stakeholders who are interested in furthering the hospital's mission. The champion understands the growth and development plan and demonstrates knowledgeable enthusiasm for the future of the hospital by communicating effectively with all interested parties. Choice *A* is incorrect because cost reduction is the responsibility of financial managers. Choice *C* is incorrect because the program champion's efforts are directed to community stakeholders rather than "in-house" employees. Choice *D* is incorrect because risk reduction team members would be responsible for investigating adverse patient-care events.

**40. A:** The most critical risk to accurate and thorough data collection is the failure to use standardized data collection measures. For example, if narrative data entry in an EHR is not well understood, then that important information may not be retrievable. Standardized measures support better communication and improve the success of quality improvement efforts. Choice *B* is incorrect because the elimination of human error is not possible. Choice *C* is incorrect because data collection methods are hospital-specific, and what is appropriate for one hospital is not necessarily the best fit for another. CMS incentives may or may not be associated with any single element of data collection; however, the incentives are not the basic requirement or initial focus of data management process planning. This means that Choice *D* is incorrect.

**41. A:** The three-fold American Hospital Association (AHA) plan is aimed at providing better care, improved population health, and lowered health care costs. One of the approaches associated with this initiative is the formation of alliances among acute care, primary care, and specialty care organizations that allow financial risk and costs to be shared across all providers. In this model, patients would receive care across the lifespan from one or more of the alliance partners as necessary. Although decreased emergency room visits might result from patient care in an alliance, the primary focus of the alliance is to share financial risk, which means that Choice *B* is incorrect. Potential revenue increases are not the alliance's focus, which means that Choice *C* is incorrect. Employee retention is not an element of the alliance criteria; therefore, Choice *D* is incorrect.

**42. B:** The process champion is most often a middle or senior level manager who promotes quality improvement and supports and mentors employees who participate in the process. The sponsor is commonly a senior-level manager who defines the specific details and requirements of the project. Choice *B* is correct because there is overlap in the roles of these group leaders, and there is often a single person responsible for both roles in a given project. The remaining roles are employee-level positions as opposed to managerial positions. The facilitator is a member of the organization who is certified as a Sigma black belt and is therefore qualified to coordinate the events of the change process and to communicate with the executive management team. Choice *A* is incorrect because in most cases, the facilitator is not a middle or senior-level manager. Choice *C* is also incorrect because the team leader manages the project and may also assume the duties of the facilitator, but the team leader would not be a senior-level manager. The scribe is responsible for maintaining a record of all team activities, and since this is an employee-level position, Choice *D* is also incorrect.

**43. B:** The healthcare system was fined for failing to blind the patient information that was added to the group websites or patient portals. The cookies attached to the websites allowed protected information to be shared with third-party analytic providers without proper notification of the patients using the sites. Patients stated that there was insufficient information for informed consent related to the use of cookies on the sites. Choice *A* is incorrect because data sharing between providers is appropriate with security protections. Choices *C* and *D* are incorrect because posting results and correcting data are not specifically related to website security.

**44. D:** All of the choices are necessary components of the priority setting process; however, the availability of resources is the delimiting factor. That means that Choices *A, B*, and *C* are incorrect because, although they are all important elements of priority setting, the availability of resources remains the highest priority.

**45. D:** Individual hospitals are required to develop and maintain a current detailed preparedness plan for likely disasters. For instance, hospitals in Boston are more likely to experience hurricanes, while hospitals in San Francisco are more likely to experience earthquakes. CMS publishes detailed checklists to assist the individual healthcare agencies but does not develop the plans. This means that Choice *A* is incorrect. The Centers for Disease Control and Prevention (CDC) issues alerts and care guidelines for specific illnesses but does not issue preparedness plans, which means that Choice *B* is incorrect. The AHA consults with the United States Department of Health and Human Services (HHS) and provides a forum for regional discussions among healthcare agencies; however, the AHA does not develop preparedness plans. Therefore, Choice *C* is incorrect.

**46. B:** The infusion pump is sensitive to pressure as the IV solution flows from the pump to the patient. This abnormal pressure can be caused by a dislodged IV catheter that allows the fluid to infiltrate the surrounding tissues, which is a critical issue. However, more frequently, the pump's alarm signals due to an IV catheter that is *positional*, which means that the alarm sounds every time a patient moves in bed. This situation can decrease the effectiveness of the alarm by delaying the staff's response to repeated alarm signals. This means that Choice *B* is correct.

The remaining choices are less commonly reported than alarm fatigue; however, the nursing staff is responsible for safe practice in each instance. Choice *A* is incorrect because although the pump interface requires the completion of a series of steps for proper function, individuals without proper training, including visitors, can input information that could result in harm to the patient. The nursing staff is responsible for checking the infusion pump for loose or frayed wiring, and all electronic equipment is routinely examined by the maintenance department. Choice *C* is incorrect because battery explosion is a rare event. The pump interface can become damaged, resulting in improper programming; however, appropriate maintenance of the pump makes this a rare occurrence as well, making Choice *D* incorrect.

**47. A:** Every group in the organization must develop an action plan that identifies how the work of the group will contribute toward the achievement of the organizational objectives. Choice *B* is incorrect because the employee action plan is also focused on how the employee's work correlates with the organizational objectives. The organizational action plan includes identification of the organizational objectives, the timelines, and those responsible for each action. Choice *C* is incorrect because the description of the action plan does not include the organization's goals or timelines. The action plans for individual groups within an organization are required to reflect the group contribution to the achievement of the organizational objectives; therefore, Choice *D* is incorrect.

**48. A:** The project charter includes all details of the quality improvement plan, including the identification of team members, planned measurement tools, and a project timeline. The plan also reflects the mission of the healthcare institution. Choice *B* is incorrect because the project charter is not a legal document; it is a planning device that is used to organize the quality improvement effort. Experts encourage the use of existing measurement tools that meet the requirements of the new project because measure development is a timely process that could negatively affect the project timeline. This means that Choice *C* is incorrect. Quality improvement projects require broad-based institutional participation for success and sustainability. Employees at all levels should be included in the process, which means that Choice *D* is incorrect.

**49. C:** The purpose of the 2016 National Strategy for Healthcare initiative is to increase the participation of the patients and families in all aspects of healthcare delivery. The expected outcome is a healthcare agency that provides affordable, safe, and patient-centered care. Improved end-of-life care may be a result of this initiative; however, it is not the primary focus. Therefore, Choice *A* is incorrect. Providers are committed to lifelong learning; however, the focus of this initiative is the involvement of the patient and family, which means that Choice *B* is incorrect. The development of IT infrastructure would support patient-centered care, but since it is not the primary goal, Choice *D* is incorrect.

**50. C:** Computer systems are password-protected, but that protection only works if the nursing staff consistently follows the protocol. An idle computer that is not secured is a breach of confidentiality and a violation of the Health Insurance Portability and Accountability Act of 1996 (HIPAA). This means that Choice *C* is the correct answer. Choice *A* is incorrect because the accuracy of data input is a form of data integrity. Choice *B* is incorrect because restricted interdepartmental sharing is an example of faulty accessibility. This problem is seen as being responsible for costly duplication of services and failure to identify possible safety risks. Choice *D* is incorrect because if patients are not able to manage the

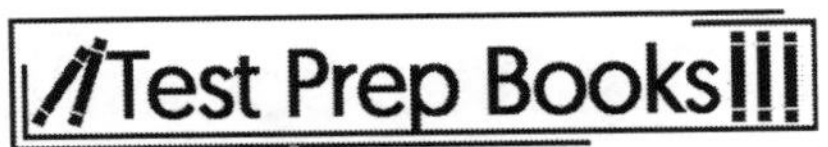

connections between the online patient resources and their devices, patient access to agency information will be decreased.

**51. C:** The assessment of quality improvement measures includes three basic forms: outcome measures that typically describe resulting behaviors in a target population, process measures that assess how the improved process is functioning, and balancing measures that add perspective to the outcome measures. Choice *C* is correct because the results of the customer satisfaction surveys put the product outcome measures in perspective. Choices *A* and *B* are incorrect because they are outcome measures that are not compared to any additional measure. Choice *D* is incorrect because it is a comparison between two outcome measures.

**52. B:** The scope of practice for licensed providers is mandated by the professional licensing board in the individual states. The leadership team must be aware of these requirements to properly credential professional providers. Choice *A* is incorrect because it describes the process of privileging, rather than credentialing. Choice *C* is incorrect because specialty certification and licensure are not generally required for all licensed providers. The leadership team can impose that requirement; however, it is beyond the definition of credentialing. The leadership team is responsible for credentialing, privileging, and oversight of licensed providers. Individual credentialing decisions are based on performance evaluations in addition to proper licensure, and not all applicants will be accepted. Therefore, Choice *D* is incorrect.

**53. D:** Special cause variations are conditions that affect the existing system. The wide range of the patients' ages is a special cause variation in the length of stay pathway because older patients would potentially present with additional co-morbidities that would affect their postoperative course. The effect of the special cause variation of patients' age could be addressed by revising the clinical pathway, the common cause variation, to reflect the situation more accurately. Choices *A, B*, and *C* are incorrect because they represent common cause variations that are inherent to the organization. The team leaders are responsible for the transfer protocol, the staffing levels and the number of available surgical suites, and common cause variations; however, team leaders do not have control over the ages of the patients.

**54. D:** Randomizing access codes and requiring agency attire increase the security of the nursing unit. Due diligence with the rules and situational awareness are essential to safe practice.

**55. D:** Indicators are measures that show the degree to which the action plan is meeting the overall objective. Choice *D* is correct because it provides a tally of the number of patients who received care. Choice *A* is incorrect because it is an overall objective of the action plan. Choice *B* is incorrect because, while it could be considered as an outcome or an output, it does include a direct measure or time frame. Choice *C* is incorrect because it is an activity used to facilitate the plan outcomes.

**56. A:** Risk management increasingly represents the relationship between financial stability and patient-care *outcomes* that can affect the entire organization. Risk management has traditionally looked to protection from liability associated with adverse events. In contrast, value-based models put the entire healthcare organization at significant financial risk because payers only reimburse patient care that meets or exceeds established outcomes. The development of diagnosis-related groups in the 1980s was aimed at the reduction of healthcare costs by using the diagnosis-related groups (DRG) codes that identified patient categories based on the patient's diagnosis, existing co-morbidities, and surgical history as the basis for payment for the care of an individual patient. This means that Choice *B* is incorrect.

Value-based care models have expanded the focus to patient-care outcomes rather than simpler patient categories such as length of stay and age. These systems affect the entire organization and are designed to promote excellent patient care with commensurate reimbursement. Fee-for-service models that pay a pre-determined fee for a specific service without regard to patient characteristics or care outcomes have been the long-standing reimbursement model that was largely eliminated with the Affordable Care Act, which means that Choice *C* is incorrect. Risk management has always been associated with potential legal costs, and that potential continues to exist in value-based care models. However, one could argue that improved patient-care outcomes could lower legal costs, which means that Choice *D* is incorrect.

**57. D:** The facilitation of a QI initiative requires an assessment of the stakeholder view, appropriate small-scale testing of the proposed change, and communication with those affected by the proposed change. Choice *D* is correct because it is an opportunity for two-way communication relative to the QI project. Choice *A* is incorrect because it is a "top-down" approach to QI. This decision-making style may be necessary for certain organizational decisions, but it is not viewed as the most productive approach to QI. Choice *B* is also incorrect because the employees were not involved in the planning or assessment of the proposed change prior to the announcement. Choice *C* is incorrect because the employees were not involved in any of the preliminary steps that led to policy changes.

**58. B:** The control chart has several functions: identifying processes for improvement, developing and implementing the new plan, evaluating the effectiveness of the plan, and monitoring the continued use of the plan over time. This means that Choices *A, C,* and *D* are incorrect. Root cause analysis is not one of the functions of the control chart.

**59. C:** The Agency for Healthcare Research and Quality (AHRQ) is a division of HHS that uses current research to develop toolkits or guidelines for the implementation of safe care practices in different care settings. TEAMSTEPPS is an organizational communication plan developed by the AHRQ and the United States Department of Defense aimed at the successful implementation of the safety recommendations. The core competencies of the AHRQ are data and analytics, healthcare research, and quality and safety improvement, which means that the agency-specific improvement plans are an essential resource for any healthcare institution. However, Choice *A* is incorrect because the AHRQ only provides the research evidence and the voluntary implementation plan. Adoption of the plan by the healthcare agency is voluntary. Choice *B* is incorrect because, as mentioned above, the AHRQ is a division of HHS and is funded by the United States government. Choice *D* is incorrect because the AHRQ maintains a comprehensive website that provides access to a wide range of resources for all researchers.

**60. B:** The instrument was developed for smaller agencies and individual practices as an aid to meeting risk assessment requirements for HIPAA and CMS, so Choice *B* is the correct answer. The assessment is required by the HIPAA Security Rule, and it is used to identify potential risks and develop a plan to mitigate those risks. Therefore, Choices *A, C,* and *D*, are incorrect.

**61. B:** The failure rate in some large organizations is as high as 60 percent. It is possible that the lack of success is due to errors in the conduct of the process rather than the process itself, which means that Choice *B* is the correct answer. Choices *A* and *C* address the expenses and training required for the implementation of the protocol. These are fixed costs that are not modifiable, which means that both

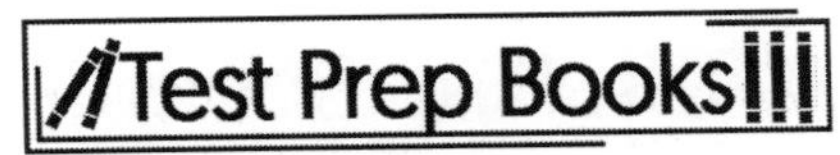

choices are incorrect. Even when the initiatives are successful, customer satisfaction is difficult to predict, which means that Choice *D* is incorrect.

**62. D:** The effectiveness of the resulting diagram depends on an accurate definition of the problem. The detailed statement is defined as the "head" of the fish, so if the statement is detailed and complete, the bones of the fish are more accurately defined.

Consider the difference between the following statements:

Problem statement: patient falls.

Problem statement: 6/24/2022 1930 sixty-six-year-old male patient was found lying on the floor. No apparent injuries.

The second statement identifies the time of day as one of the issues that would not necessarily be identified in the first statement. The fall occurred during the change of shift, which would then be one of the "bones" on the diagram. The team members do not all have to be quality improvement experts; however, the team members should be knowledgeable about the process as well as the problem being discussed. This means that Choice *A* is incorrect. Human error is commonly identified by root cause analysis in healthcare, but identifying human error is not the primary purpose of the model. So, Choice *B* is incorrect. Punitive action is contrary to the purpose of quality improvement, which is better patient care. This means that Choice *C* is incorrect.

**63. B:** The Institute for Healthcare Improvement (IHI) is a private non-profit organization that is partially funded by grants from the AHRQ. The focus of the IHI is the worldwide implementation of safe patient-care practices. The Science of Improvement is based on identifying areas for improvement and testing new ideas according to the plan, do, study, act (PDSA) sequence rather than error analysis. This means that Choice *A* is incorrect. Implementation of IHI improvement plans is voluntary and not associated with CMS reimbursement, so Choice *C* is incorrect. The IHI improvement plans apply to all patient-care environments, which means that Choice *D* is incorrect.

**64. A:** Pareto analysis identifies the areas that require intervention; however, identification of the costs associated with the proposed actions is not addressed in the analysis. The remaining activities are included in the Pareto model, which means that Choices *B, C,* and *D* are incorrect.

**65. A:** High-reliability organizations are complex systems with inherent risk potential that function without reported errors for extended periods. This means that Choice *A* is correct. Choice *B* is incorrect because system processes are streamlined but not simplified; simplification can potentially hide risks associated with the process. Choice *C* is incorrect because "deference to expertise" is one of the identified characteristics, which means that every individual in the system is an expert in their work and is therefore responsible for risk reduction. Choice *D* is incorrect because near-misses are viewed as system failures that identify areas for improvement rather than successes.

**66. D:** The National Quality Forum (NQF) is a non-profit, non-partisan research foundation that develops measurement tools for safe practice evaluation in multiple care settings. For instance, if a hospital implements a new protocol for surgical site wound care, an NQF measure could be used to evaluate and report the outcomes of that new protocol. CMS consults with the Measure Applications Partnership, a division of NQF, to provide measures that accurately reflect an agency's healthcare quality. Choice *A* is incorrect because the NQF is funded by donors. Choice *B* is incorrect because the NQF develops evaluation measures rather than communication plans. Choice *C* is incorrect because the NQF includes a wide range of stakeholders, including patients, measurement experts, and healthcare professionals, in the development of the evaluation measures.

**67. C:** Root cause analysis categorizes causes as physical, human, or organizational. Choice *C* is correct because the cause of the discrepancy was directly related to the failure of the institution to identify the proper protocol for controlled substance reconciliation. Choice *A* is a human issue because only a single licensed person verified the count when two signatures were necessary, which means that Choice *A* is incorrect. Choice *B* is incorrect because the computer malfunction is a physical cause. Choice *D* also describes a human cause, so it too is incorrect.

**68. C:** Risk-adjustment methods are mathematical projections of the care costs for a population of patients based on demographics and diagnoses, which are beyond the control of the provider. The models are used for CMS and third-party payer reimbursement. Choice *A* is incorrect because the development of the models was commissioned by CMS in the 1990s as a provider reimbursement framework. The projections and the reimbursement rates are now published annually by CMS. As noted, the models adjust outcomes for demographic status and medical diagnoses, which means that Choice *B* is incorrect. The risk models are also used by third-party payers to set rates for enrollees, so that means that Choice *D* is incorrect.

**69. B:** The CATWOE assessment is designed to assess business priorities from the customers' view. Additional elements are assessed; however, the primary focus is on the customer base, which means that Choice *B* is correct. Cause and effect analysis identifies every possible issue that might affect business outcomes. Choice *A* is incorrect because the primary focus of this measure is not limited to customer preferences. Risk analysis identifies all issues that may present as vulnerabilities or issues that might affect business outcomes. Although customer satisfaction could affect business outcomes, it is not the only issue considered with this measure; therefore, Choice *C* is incorrect. Impact analysis identifies the potential effects of natural disasters or other emergencies. This measure does not assess customer satisfaction, so Choice *D* is incorrect.

**70. A:** The World Health Organization (WHO) is a division of the United Nations that is charged with overseeing worldwide health concerns. WHO focuses on the dissemination and use of research aimed at a wide range of issues from infectious disease control to the health effects of climate change. Choice *B* is incorrect because WHO decisions can be and are challenged by member nations. Choice *C* is incorrect because WHO provides practice guidelines for infectious diseases but does not provide case management for individuals with the disease. WHO provides worldwide alerts regarding infectious diseases; however, WHO is not responsible for the actual development of vaccines. Therefore, Choice *D* is incorrect.

**71. A:** The scatter diagram is used to display pairs of numerical data. In the example, patient age groups and the number of clinic visits would be compared and displayed. The fishbone diagram is used to determine cause and effect, which means that Choice *B* is incorrect. The control chart is a detailed time-series view of an entire process, which tracks changes over time. Choice *C* is incorrect because the question does not specify a time-series model. The Pareto chart estimates the impact of multiple factors on outcome measures, which means that Choice *D* is incorrect; the example only requires the relationship between one pair of variables.

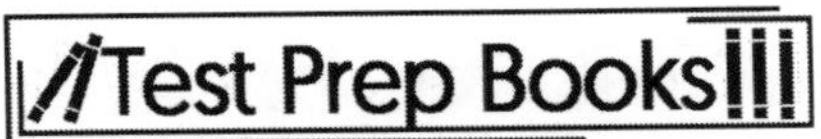

**72. A:** The purpose of the process control measurement is to prevent errors from reaching the customer. These measures should be identified for each possible cause identified in the FMEA analysis; therefore, Choice *A* is correct. Choice *B* is incorrect because identifying links is more common in a cause-and-effect study. The process control would not apply to employee performance criteria, which means that Choice *C* is incorrect. A time and motion study could ultimately affect customer satisfaction, but the focus is on the production of the product, so Choice *D* is incorrect.

**73. C:** Patient care visits that are canceled and not rescheduled often result in poor patient outcomes. The delay in rescheduling the appointment means that any changes in the patient's condition will be untreated for a longer period, and the patient's questions and concerns will not be addressed. Therefore, Choice *C* is the correct answer. Loss of revenue, staffing issues, and CMS reporting criteria are all significant issues related to cancelled appointments that are not rescheduled. However, the greatest risk is poor patient outcomes resulting from sub-standard care.

**74. C:** Healthcare Effectiveness Data and Information Set (HEDIS) databases, a product of the National Committee for Quality Assurance (NCQA), are intended to provide a comprehensive evaluation of the effectiveness of healthcare plans. The NCQA determines performance standards for six domains of care including effectiveness, access and availability of care, patient-care experiences, health-plan utilization and descriptive data, and the use of the Electronic Healthcare Record (EHR) for clinical data reporting. The HEDIS databases provide a comparison of established performance standards with performance data voluntarily submitted by individual healthcare plans.

This comparison provides the healthcare plan administrators with the identification of areas requiring improvement and also provides consumers with a reliable resource for comparing healthcare plans. Choice *A* is incorrect because the HEDIS database is used to evaluate healthcare plan effectiveness, not communicable disease tracking. Choice *B* is incorrect because the evaluation of environmental services would not be evaluated in the healthcare plan assessment. CMS has contracted with NCQA to establish performance standards for Special Needs Plans (SNPs) to be added to the performance evaluation of the healthcare plans. For instance, an SNP was developed to evaluate the plan's performance in medication reconciliation after hospital discharge. The performance standard would evaluate when and how the medication check was completed. Choice *D* is incorrect because the EHR use would be evaluated for accuracy of the medication list, patient access to the list, and verification of the post-discharge medication check.

**75. D:** Choice *D* is the correct answer because it is not objectively measurable. The remaining choices are incorrect because it is possible to assess each of the process champion's performances objectively. Choice *A* is incorrect because the relationship between the process champion and the patient can be measured objectively. Team members can report on the effectiveness of the process champion as a leader, which means that Choice *B* is incorrect. Choice *C* is incorrect because it is possible to measure the relationships between the process champions, senior management, and team members.

**76. D:** The point of ERM is that every aspect of a single healthcare system must be subject to ongoing critical analysis of risk potential. This whole-system approach doesn't deviate from an emphasis on patient outcomes, but rather expands the scope of risk analysis to include every circumstance that could affect patient outcomes; therefore, Choice *D* is the correct answer. Choices *A* and *C* are more recent additions to risk assessment models, and Choice *B* has always been addressed in the risk assessment models.

**77. B:** A structural measure provides patients with information about the provider that can affect care choices. The number of board-certified providers is generally accepted as a measure of quality, which would be an important addition to the marketing strategy. Choice *A* is incorrect because glaucoma screening for all patients over forty-five years old would be a process measure. The screening affects the health of a patient population. Choices *C* and *D* are incorrect because they are outcome measures that reflect the quality of care.

**78. B:** When rates of innovation adoption by a group are plotted on a bell curve, the early adopters are 13.5 percent of the entire group. This group identifies the pros and cons of the proposed innovation and then decides to adopt the solution. Group leaders are most often identified as early adopters based on their assessment of the value of the innovation rather than on the "newness" of the innovation (innovators), or the need to "wait and see" how it works (majority). Choice *A* is incorrect because diffusion is often a slow process, even for changes that are widely anticipated. Choice *C* is incorrect because late majority adopters are slow to recognize the value of the innovation, and more commonly take a "wait and see" attitude before adopting the changes. Choice *D* is incorrect because the diffusion of an idea in a social system can occur informally without deliberate dissemination by system leaders.

**79. C:** Risk management provides value to a business, but the customer is not going to pay for it. That is the definition of a business value-added activity, which means that Choice *C* is correct. Choice *A* is incorrect because meeting government regulations is a required non-value-added activity. Choice *B* is incorrect because accommodating contracted customer requirements is a non-value-added activity. Choice *D* is a non-value-added activity that is considered a waste by Sigma standards.

**80. C:** Situation awareness means planning for "what if." The handoff report alerts the oncoming nurse to the possible development of pneumonia, which could be confirmed with a chest x-ray. This means that Choice *C* is correct. Choice *A* is incorrect because it provides a timeline and important information about the patient's condition for the oncoming nurse. Choice *B* is incorrect because it describes the patient's illness stability. Choice *D* is incorrect because it is an example of synthesis, or "talk back" in which the oncoming nurse repeats the summary.

**81. A:** Disease management is a form of case management that constructs a care plan for patients with largely predictable outcomes. The elderly female patient who has a knee arthroplasty generally follows a predictable course that facilitates care planning. The remaining choices are incorrect because the diagnoses are either potentially evolving or are at least unpredictable. Hemorrhagic strokes and posterior wall MIs can extend, and tumor lysis syndrome can produce unpredictable effects, which means that Choices *B, C,* and *D* are incorrect.

**82. D:** The Pareto chart is used to identify areas for potential quality improvement. It is based on the 80/20 rule, which states that 80 percent of the effect is due to 20 percent of the causes. For instance, if the team identifies ten common patient complaints, the 80/20 principle predicts that 80 percent of the patient complaints are related to only two of the identified complaints. The Control Charts or Run Charts examine variation; however, the Pareto chart cannot identify either common cause or special cause variation effects. This means that Choice *A* is incorrect. The Pareto chart is relevant for the initial quality improvement planning; however, the resulting data can also be used in the analysis and evaluation phases to assess the continued success of the innovations. This means that Choice *B* is incorrect. The Pareto chart only measures variables on the categorical, nominal, or ordinal level, which means that Choice *C* is incorrect.

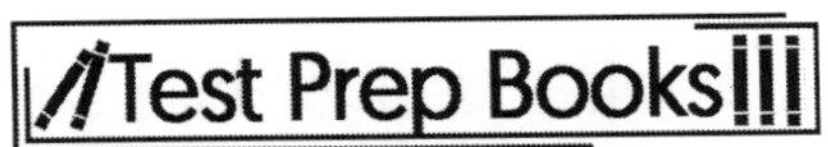

**83. A:** A fluctuation in environmental conditions is identified as a common cause variation that is expected and acceptable, which means that Choice *A* is correct. The remaining choices are incorrect because they are all special cause variations that are unexpected and not acceptable.

**84. A:** The IPASS mnemonic stands for the following: illness severity (I), patient information (P), action list (A), situational awareness and contingency plans (S), and synthesis by the receiver (S). The patient experiencing chest pain is unstable, which is the first element of the IPASS report. There are additional details related to the patient's pain that will be reported in subsequent sections of the protocol; for example, the patient's medication history or EKG patterns will be reported in the patient summary (P) or the to-do list (A). However, the critical element will be reported first. This means that Choices *B, C,* and *D* are incorrect.

**85. B:** The 5 Whys focuses on identifying the root cause as opposed to a solution that may or may not provide long-term improvement in the situation. Choice *A* is incorrect because the purpose of the technique is to solve the problem. Choice *C* is incorrect because there is no certainty that countermeasures or solutions would be less difficult to implement. The team charged with using the 5 Whys technique does not require management approval of the identified countermeasures, which means that Choice *D* is incorrect.

**86. A:** Three choices define illness severity in the I-PASS model: stable, watcher, or unstable. The watcher category includes patients that require close observation because their conditions have inherent risk. For example, the patient being treated for atrial fibrillation with anticoagulant therapy has a risk of bleeding, and the patient with a mild cognitive deficit has increased safety issues. The stable category includes patients who require routine monitoring that is appropriate to their condition, and the unstable category includes patients who require emergency management. This means that Choice *A* is correct. Choice *B* is incorrect because it describes a timeline according to the mnemonic. Choices *C* and *D* each describe situation awareness, looking ahead at possible patient needs.

**87. B:** Registries are databases that focus on a single disease, condition, or patient characteristic for research purposes related to treatment effectiveness, tracking of implanted devices in case of product recalls, or comparing the patient-care outcomes of different healthcare organizations. Choice *A* is incorrect because failure to share data between systems is one of the most critical shortcomings of current EHR systems. Capturing care costs is a routine function of the EHR system and the information would not be included in a patient-specific registry, which means that Choice *C* is incorrect. Registries are focused on patient data for improved patient care, which means that Choice *D* is incorrect.

**88. A:** The CMS Meaningful Measures 2022 initiative is focused on identifying areas for quality improvement and providing a comprehensive list of assessment measures. The remaining choices may be addressed in individual measures included in the list; however, the focus of the initiative is the identification of both the healthcare issue and the assessment measures. That means that Choices *B, C,* and *D* are incorrect.

**89. C:** Scorecards and dashboards are both used to identify data that require additional action by the hospital. Experts argue that unused data shouldn't be collected. Scorecards are a detailed long-term picture of the strategic plan for the organization. The scorecards are used by senior managers for institutional-level evaluation and planning. In contrast, dashboards are real-time measures of systems operations that are used by frontline managers to direct workflow. Choice *A* is incorrect because scorecards address the long-term strategic view of the organization rather than the identification of a single quality improvement effort. Dashboards address the issues associated with the real-time performance of process and outcome measures, which means that Choice *B* is incorrect. Drill-down capability means that the data-entry system allows current data to be instantly connected to comparative or historical data. Scorecards that take the long-term view do not require this capability; however, this function is a requirement for dashboards that are used for real-time comparisons by the frontline managers. This means that Choice *D* is incorrect.

**90. C:** Direct messages are the best indicator of the conversions for that site. Conversions are defined as the number of people who visit the site and become customers. Likes, follows, and social shares indicate different levels of engagement with the product or the corporation; however, the conversion rates from website viewer to paying customer are lower than the direct messaging metric. This means that Choices *A*, *B*, and *D* are incorrect.

**91. B:** Two HIPAA safeguards address access to PHI. Audit controls track access to PHI over time while access controls identify the procedures that restrict access to PHI. Integrity controls refer to procedures that protect PHI from unauthorized edits or data loss, which means that Choice *A* is incorrect. Choice *C* is incorrect because transmission security refers to the protection of PHI that is sent to another device, such as sending data by email to another provider.

**92. C:** The thirty-day readmission rate is a long-term measure that would be checked as an element of strategic planning, which is consistent with the use of the scorecard by senior management. Choices *A*, *B*, and *D* are measures used in real-time by frontline managers, which means that these choices are incorrect.

**93. D:** The IHI initiative was a response to the Institute of Medicine (IOM)'s earlier reports of widespread errors and inequities in healthcare in the United States. The primary interest of the IHI initiative was improved quality of care for all patients (including timeliness, effectiveness, and efficiency) rather than cost containment. That means that Choices *A*, *B*, and *C* are incorrect.

**94: B**: Choice *B* is correct because ISO 9000 focuses on production standards, but it does not include any assessment of the finished product's quality. ISO 9000 standards do address the importance of stakeholder involvement in terms of client satisfaction and proper use of employee talent and expertise, which means that Choices *A* and *C* are incorrect. Senior management's approval and support are essential to the successful use of this product improvement framework; therefore, Choice *D* is incorrect.

**95. B**: Non-probability sampling methods are prone to bias and do not use random assignment. Probability sampling methods require random sampling of some form designed to eliminate or limit bias. This means that Choice *A* is incorrect. Voluntary sampling does not include any form of random assignment, which is required for probability sampling; therefore, Choice *C* is incorrect. Non-probability sampling methods do not include random assignment, which means that Choice *D* is incorrect.

**96. C:** The time from the decision to admit an ER patient to the patient's arrival on the nursing unit is a reportable Electronic Clinical Quality Measure (eCQM) that demonstrates quality care. Choice *A* is incorrect because the actual measure assesses the number of infants who are *breastfed* from birth to discharge, which is evidence of the quality of patient education related to the importance of breastfeeding. Choice *B* is also incorrect because the eCQMs are measures of patient-care quality that would be expressed as a positive outcome (e.g., an eCQM might be the number of non-ambulatory

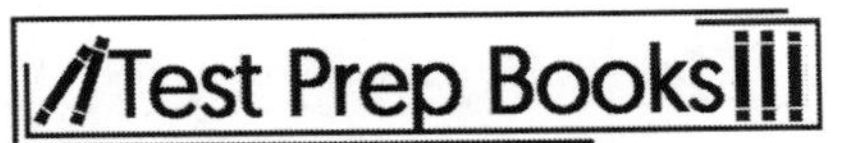

patients with documentation of skin assessment every shift). Choice *D* is incorrect because opioid documentation is mandatory and must be submitted in addition to the voluntary reports.

**97: A:** Choice *A* is correct because Lean is focused on removing wastes, which are also described as non-value-added activities. Lean uses simpler methods such as reorganization of the production process workplace analysis techniques such as the 5 Whys while Six Sigma employs hypothesis testing; therefore, Choice *B* is incorrect. Six Sigma is focused on process variation while Lean is focused on waste reduction, which means that Choice *C* is incorrect. Choice *D* is incorrect because Lean is the suggested first step in process improvement; progression to Six Sigma analysis occurs as needed depending on the situation.

**98. D:** The most frequent issues associated with imported data sources are formatting problems. Hospital managers must assess all aspects of the imported data for errors. Authoritative data sources that meet the needs of the hospital plan would be expected to be bias-free, which means that Choice *A* is incorrect. The costs of data analysis vary according to the specific needs and resources of the organization, which means that Choice *B* is incorrect. Experts caution hospitals to examine the data before the creation of objects such as tables and graphs due to the possible effects of inaccurate information. Therefore, Choice *C* is incorrect.

**99. C:** The Employee Net Promoter Scale (eNPS) identifies employees as more or less satisfied with their position in the company. The scale uses the responses to a single question to categorize respondents as promoters, passives, or detractors, depending on the likelihood that the individual would recommend their company as a good place to work. The remaining choices are incorrect because they are not included in or have no relevance to the scale.

**100. A:** Cyber experts voice concerns about the level of protection afforded by compliance with HIPAA standards. The weakness lies in the cyber security levels of the healthcare system's business associates such as vendors and primary care partners. For instance, if the security of the All-Care Primary Practice is less than secure, breaches of that system can extend to the General Hospital system, and that potential risk is not addressed in the HIPAA security standards. Therefore, Choice *A* is correct. Choice *B* is incorrect because the critical issue in cyber security is the need for continuous surveillance for gaps and initiation of protection updates. Choice *C* is incorrect because all systems are vulnerable to cyber breaches and protection against the threats is a continuous process. Choice *D* is incorrect because two-factor authorization (2FA) is considered the minimum standard and multi-factor authorization is the preferred (MFA) standard for all partner systems that interface with the hospital system.

**101. A:** Benchmarks may be imposed externally by JCAHO and CMS, or they may be identified by senior managers for internal monitoring. Effective benchmarking depends on input from a broad range of stakeholders. Senior managers can identify benchmarks for internal audits in addition to the benchmark reports required by JCAHO and CMS. This means that Choices *B* and *C* are incorrect. Benchmarking is required for all healthcare facilities that are reimbursed by CMS, which means that Choice *D* is incorrect.

**102. A:** The sale of the protected health information (PHI) is consistent with the intent of the most severe criminal offense because the PHI was accessed under false pretenses, and the staff member intended to sell the information for personal gain. Choice *B* is also a criminal violation because the information was accessed without a "need to know." This violation is also commonly associated with agency dismissal rather than a prison sentence. The nursing assistant's error described in Choice *C* would be considered a civil violation related to lack of knowledge rather than criminal intent, which means that Choice *C* is incorrect. Choice *D* is an example of a civil violation identified as willful neglect. The nurse was aware of the correct procedure; however, these violations are not assessed penalties if the violation is corrected within thirty days of the occurrence. In this instance, the hospital might be required to schedule additional information sessions, or the IT department might be required to modify the default "timeout" for active patient pages in the hospital's EHR system. This means that Choice *D* is incorrect.

**103. C:** By definition, an external-helpful factor would be something that benefits the organization but is not under its control. That means that Choice *C* is correct because the funds are beneficial to the organization, but the organization did not have control over the award of the benefit. Existing organizational resources would be considered a helpful benefit; however, the control would be internal rather than external, which means that Choice *A* is incorrect. Knowledge gained from past failures is regarded as internal and helpful as well, so Choice *B* is incorrect. Losing customers due to supply chain issues would be an external-unhelpful factor because the loss is detrimental and not controlled by the organization, which means that Choice *D* is incorrect.

**104. D:** Conflicts and lack of cooperation between departments in a healthcare system are viewed as socio-organizational environmental barriers in the PETT model. Choices *A* and *B* are incorrect because they are identified as people issues in the model. Choice *C* is also incorrect because the model considers the complex interface as a tool, and it is a barrier when people find it difficult to use.

**105. B:** Meaningful Use criteria address the use of the EHR in three specific areas that include providing a tangible patient service such as e-prescribing, facilitating the electronic exchange of information between providers or healthcare systems, and communicating the quality-of-care indicators. Financial schedules for reimbursement of any service are not included in the Meaningful Use criteria because the criteria are focused on the direct enhancement of the patient's care experience. The use of the EHR for e-prescribing can positively affect the patient's experience, which means that Choice *A* is incorrect. The patient's care experience and engagement in the treatment plan are positively affected by using an EHR system that can successfully share information with another system. This means that Choice *C* is incorrect. EHR systems that can be used to transmit the quality-of-care data such as A1C results meet the third Meaningful Use objective; therefore, Choice *D* is incorrect.

**106. C:** The most common "ribs" of the fishbone diagram are materials, methods, equipment, environment, and people. The model is focused on identifying the root cause of an error by tracking the information associated with these categories. This means that Choices *A, B,* and *D* are incorrect because they are classic categories associated with the model.

**107. D:** The Agile philosophy is based on the importance of close collaboration with the customer at each step of the process, which means that Choice *D* is the correct answer. The Agile program is commonly used by software developers who often deliver a workable prototype to the customer in the early stages of the design process. That model then provides the basis for the design changes going forward. This means that Choice *A* is incorrect. In addition, customer-generated revisions are encouraged and welcomed at any point in the process, which means that Choice *B* is also incorrect. Social media may be used to maintain contact with the customer base; however, the most common marketing strategy associated with this model is face-to-face interaction. This means that Choice *C* is incorrect.

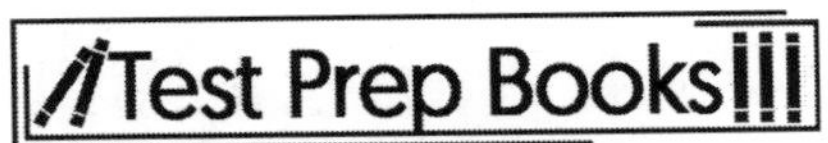

**108. D:** State licensing boards in thirty-seven states restrict physicians from telehealth visits across state lines; however, there were accommodations made by most states during the COVID-19 pandemic. Currently, some states are again requiring licensure in the state where the care is provided. For instance, during the pandemic, a physician in New Jersey could provide telehealth care for a patient in Connecticut. Presently, both states have rescinded those rules and reverted to the pre-pandemic requirements for MD licensure in the state where the care was rendered. The remaining states have either accepted temporary waiver applications or adopted the alternative licensure rules.

Nurse licensure rules also vary from state to state. Except for California, Oregon, Nevada, and Hawaii, the states have established compact licensure, which allows a nurse registered in a "compact" state to work in another compact state without obtaining a license in the second state.

Choice *A* is incorrect because the main issue with technology is sufficient funding, which would not affect interstate delivery of care. Choice *B* is incorrect because software licensing is between the developer and the healthcare agency rather than the geographic scope of practice. Choice *C* is incorrect because Medicaid payments are set by the states while Medicare payments are set by CMS.

**109. A:** The clan culture is characterized by a collaborative work environment wherein each person has a voice. This model is associated with happy and involved employees, which promotes the growth of the new company; therefore, Choice *A* is correct. Adhocracy culture is defined by its vision and is characteristic of companies that set the pace for innovation in the marketplace. Choice *B* is incorrect because a start-up company would rarely achieve this standing in the marketplace. The hierarchy culture is defined as the traditional top-down structure that is focused on internal control and avoidance of risk. These characteristics would be counter-productive for a start-up company; therefore, Choice *C* is incorrect. Choice *D* is incorrect because the market culture focuses on external successes rather than the creation of a happy workforce that is characteristic of start-up companies.

**110. A:** Multi-stage sampling is a form of cluster sampling that samples large populations efficiently. Stratified sampling is used effectively with homogenous groups, which means that Choice *B* is incorrect. Bias can only be statistically controlled, not eliminated, with random sampling, which means that Choice *C* is incorrect. There are no sample size requirements for multi-stage sampling, so Choice *D* is incorrect.

**111. C:** The theory suggests that praising small steps toward the desired behavior increases the rate of change and success of the desired behavior. Choice *A* is incorrect because the group must have a workable strategy in place to identify possible barriers. The members of the coalition must include all stakeholders to promote effective change. The group will include senior management; however, staff members, patients, and families must also be included as appropriate. This means that Choice *B* is incorrect. Communicating the vision must occur before any change can be expected. Individuals affected by the proposed changes must see the need for the change, or at least agree that some form of change is required, which means that Choice *D* is incorrect.

**112. B:** In a company with a hierarchical culture, employee-level decisions would most likely occur at the operational planning stage, which involves the identification of project standards and work schedules. In the hierarchical culture model, contingency, tactical, and strategic planning would be the responsibility of mid-level managers rather than the employees, which means that Choices *A, C,* and *D* are incorrect.

**113. C:** The Hospital Readmissions Reduction Program (HRRP) is an incentive program that assesses penalties for poor performance on the 30-day readmission measures for several diagnoses that are commonly associated with readmission. Improved communication, especially at the point of discharge, is one of the ways that hospitals can decrease readmission rates. Improved communication between the hospitals and providers results in an effective care plan that can prevent early readmission. The most common conditions are heart failure, myocardial infarction, chronic obstructive pulmonary disease (COPD), post-operative joint replacement, and hospital-acquired infections such as pneumonia. The plan applies to patients covered by Medicare, not Medicaid, which means that Choice *A* is incorrect. End-stage renal disease costs are not addressed in this measure, so Choice *B* is incorrect. Patient education is not addressed in this measure, which means that Choice *D* is incorrect.

**114. B:** High-reliability healthcare systems (HROs) demonstrate resiliency by using errors that occur to shape mitigation plans for the next untoward event, which means that Choice *B* is correct. HROs also defer to the expertise of the individual closest to the task to identify risks and mitigation strategies for that process, which refers to the HRO characteristic of deference to expertise, which means that Choice *A* is incorrect. In addition, the employees are provided with the appropriate educational resources, and they have a strong voice in risk management activities. These choices relate to the HRO characteristics that include sensitivity to operations, which means that Choices *C* and *D* are incorrect.

**115. C:** The virtual private network (VPN) masks the hospital's internal information while protecting against unauthorized access to the system. The use of the VPN meets HIPPA regulations and facilitates the safe transfer of PHI. The VPN provides a password-protected email system for the entire organization rather than only senior managers, which means that Choice *A* is incorrect. A VPN would not be required to support a remote position or to stream patient teaching modules, so Choices *B* and *D* are incorrect.

**116. B:** Even though the United States spends more than twice as much money on healthcare than other developed nations, healthcare outcome measures are worse and life expectancy is shorter. CMS is moving to a value-based reimbursement plan to address rising costs and declining quality of care. Providers are advised to identify and measure the effectiveness of KPIs such as hospital readmission rates, patient satisfaction, and ER visits as evidence of the quality of care. The financial risk assumed by the provider varies with the design of the value-based care model used by the practice. There are three basic models that include the Accountable Care Organizations, Bundled Payment plans, and the Patient-Centered Medical Home model, and each model assumes some but not all of the financial risks; therefore, Choice *A* is incorrect. Value-based modifiers address provider care, not hospital care, which means that Choices *C* and *D* are incorrect.

**117. A**: Choice *A* is correct because the valley stream map traces the availability of all required resources at each step in the process. The map is also used to identify wastes or redundancies in the process. The basic flow sheet is useful at the beginning of the project to provide an overall view; however, the chart does not assess the availability of resources, which means that Choice *B* is incorrect. Choice *C* is incorrect because, while the value chain map is focused on identifying the steps of a process, it is not designed to track the availability of resources or to identify areas of waste. The cross functional map identifies connections among the processes and the people. The map identifies what resources are required; however, it does not document the availability of the resources. That means that Choice *D* is incorrect.

**118. C:** Value-based care models are associated with financial risk for the provider. Generally speaking, upside risk means that if the provider meets the patient-care goals set by CMS or a private payer, the provider shares the savings with the payer, and downside risk means that the provider is penalized for

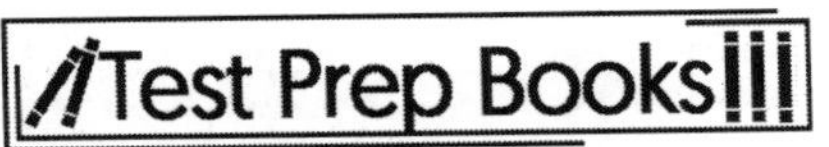

failing to meet the patient-care goals. Although there are greater rewards for quality patient care by providers in models with downside risk, many providers, especially groups that include hospitals, are not joining these models.

CMS saves more money with downside risk models and for that reason, it is currently promoting participation in hybrid, or two-sided, risk models that limit participation in models with only upside risk. Providers that participate in a downside risk model such as the Medical Home must be well coordinated to avoid the penalties associated with the model. Choice *A* is incorrect because upside risk is not associated with penalties for failure to meet metrics. CMS benefits from the penalties associated with downside risk models and would not limit provider participation in the model, which means that Choice *B* is incorrect. Downside risk models are associated with penalties for care outcomes that do not meet CMS standards, which means that Choice *D* is incorrect.

**119. B:** Stratified sampling is designed to increase sampling efficiency, which is a measure of the quality and amount of data obtained from the analysis. The sampling strata must contain mutually exclusive groups of participants, while the contents of the individual stratum should be homogenous. The homogeneity of the individual stratum decreases the variability of the sampling results, which improves the quality of the data analysis. Stratified sampling has greater sampling efficiency than random sampling due to the homogeneity of the individual stratum and the contrast between the mutually exclusive groups. This means that Choice *A* is incorrect. Volunteer sampling is a non-probability method that is not part of stratified sampling, which means that Choice *C* is incorrect. Stratified sampling is not dependent on sample size, which means that Choice *D* is incorrect.

**120. D:** BPM requires a continuous exploration of processes in an organization, especially those important processes that exist only in the heads of the people who developed and used the process. BPM focuses on the identification, evaluation, and appropriate implementation of all organizational processes that affect outcomes, which means that Choice *D* is correct. BPM is an organizational philosophy of continuous evaluation of processes that is shared with employees and management; therefore, Choice *A* is incorrect. BPM relies on the ability of the Business Process Champion to look to the future and communicate that plan to the entire organization. The Business Process Champion looks forward rather than backward, which means that Choice *B* is incorrect. The success of BPM is enhanced by team members who can employ the principles of Six Sigma; therefore, Choice *C* is incorrect.

**121. D:** Control charts provide a time-series view of system processes that highlights areas for improvement. The chart tracks process and outcomes measures; however, structural measures are not included in that chart, so Choice *A* is incorrect. Stable processes often indicate areas for improvement such as increasing the performance benchmark for a process. For instance, if the nursing staff is meeting the benchmark for 80 percent documentation of the use of the IV infusion, that process should be re-evaluated and improved to meet a higher benchmark. This means that Choice *B* is incorrect. One of the purposes of the control chart is to identify the effects of special cause variations on system processes, which means that Choice *C* is incorrect.

**122. A:** Choice *A* is correct because it is the outcome measure of Choices *B, C*, and *D*. Readmission rates for high-risk diagnoses such as chronic heart failure have been positively associated with attention to patient education, medication management, and comprehensive post-discharge care. This means that Choices *B, C*, and *D* are incorrect.

**123. B:** A mission statement is more concrete than a vision statement, and it is less precise than goals and objectives. Providing a quality product is a broad statement that includes more specific details than the mission statement, which means that Choice *B* is correct. Choice *A* is incorrect because it is a vision statement that broadly defines the reason that the company exists. Choice *C* is a goal that is timed and measurable, and more specific than a mission statement. That means that Choice *C* is incorrect. The eighty-twenty rule is a measure of variances that are used when determining the action plan and it is not related to the mission statement; therefore, Choice *D* is incorrect.

**124. B:** The Enterprise Application software addresses the data management requirements for hospital-wide processes such as OSHA compliance rather than individual patient-care outcomes. The Reliability Centered Maintenance (RCM) system evaluates risks associated with equipment costs and maintenance, which means that Choice *A* is incorrect. The EHR effectiveness surveys and the HCRM survey are patient-specific records that do not track compliance with system-wide measures, so Choices *C* and *D* are incorrect.

**125. D:** Economists suggest that integrating social services with healthcare interventions will decrease overall care costs. The plan proposes that federal funding of all Medicaid patients should be contingent upon the enrollment of covered patients in appropriate social services such as Head Start, nutritional support, and housing assistance. The major change is the federal funding of the plan for all Medicaid patients, rather than Medicare patients. This means that Choice *A* is incorrect. Choices *B* and *C* are incorrect because the unique part of the plan is applying the changes to federal funding of all Medicaid patients, rather than reporting patient data.

# Practice Test #3

1. One of the hallmarks of the value-based models is increased patient and family engagement. Which of the following values is associated with the CMS Patient and Family Engagement Strategy?
    a. Health literacy
    b. Equity
    c. Transparency
    d. Accessibility

2. The diabetic clinic staff nurses are reviewing the HbA1C results for a patient. The results are 4.8, 5.3, 6.5, 4.7, 5.3, 6.3, and 5.3. What is the mode for this group of results?
    a. 5.3
    b. 5.5
    c. 6.3
    d. 4.7

3. A team is using the RACI model to track the responsible party for each task of a proposed project. The acronym stands for "responsible, accountable, consulted, and informed." Which of the following definitions is correct?
    a. The responsible person will be a manager.
    b. The accountable person will perform the work.
    c. The consulted person will be a team member.
    d. The informed person will approve the completed work.

4. Transition-of-care errors are frequently associated with inadequate or ineffective patient information resources. Which of the following is consistent with the goals of the organizational health literacy strategies?
    a. Increasing online bill payments
    b. Improving vaccination tracking
    c. Improving patient engagement
    d. Increasing online patient feedback

5. In Tuckman's forming stage, what is the general demeanor of the team members?
    a. Competitive
    b. Agreeable
    c. Motivated
    d. Frustrated

6. Which of the following choices is consistent with statistical process control (SPC) measures?
    a. Quality improvement principles dictate the details of the SPC measure.
    b. SPC results can prove the effectiveness of the quality improvement interventions.
    c. The SPC measures are not sensitive to spontaneous variations.
    d. The measures identify the common cause and special cause variations.

7. RN staffing levels are related to patient satisfaction. The American Nurses Association (ANA) has identified issues that affect this relationship. Under non-pandemic conditions, which of the issues is under the direct control of the organizational leaders?
   a. The number of daily admissions and discharges
   b. Technical resources and support
   c. Average patient acuity level
   d. The number of patient beds in the unit

8. Which stage of Tuckman's model is the most challenging for the leader?
   a. Forming
   b. Storming
   c. Norming
   d. Performing

9. Which of the following is consistent with trend analysis?
   a. Trends are automatically generated in a time-series analysis.
   b. The trend pattern may be repeated during the measurement time.
   c. Trends represent changes in a factor or process over time.
   d. Time-series trends are always linear.

10. Healthcare delivery errors can result in a sentinel event or a near-miss event. Which of the following is consistent with a sentinel event?
   a. The sentinel event wasn't reported before the effects were discovered.
   b. The error resulted in actual physical harm to one or more individuals.
   c. Sentinel events are organizational-level errors.
   d. The error was associated with potential harm only.

11. Which of the following activities is part of the third and final phase of the Meaningful Use Initiative?
   a. Transmitting new cases of cancer to the state registry
   b. Submitting state-required immunization data
   c. Reporting lab results to state agencies
   d. Transmitting new prescription requests

12. A team is using failure mode and effect analysis (FMEA) to assess the prototype for an IV infusion pump. If each of the identified defects listed below were scored on a scale of 1-10 for effect on the customer, how often it occurs, and how obvious the defect is, which defect would receive the highest score?
   a. The electrical cord is difficult to attach.
   b. The "mL per hour" numerals are not visible in low light.
   c. The alarm volume cannot be adjusted.
   d. The prototype pump weighs one pound more than the previous model.

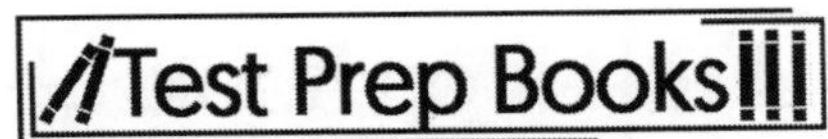

13. Transition-of-care errors have prompted the development of the Five-Star Quality Rating System by CMS. Healthcare plans are rated on a scale of one to five points according to their performance on four transition measures. Which of the following measures is NOT included in the Quality Rating documentation?
   a. Primary care provider notification of admission
   b. Patient vaccination history
   c. Medication reconciliation on or before the face-to-face visit
   d. Face-to-face "patient engagement" within 30 days of discharge

14. What is the effect of using the median value in place of the mean value in data analysis?
   a. Data trends are automatically identified.
   b. Outlier effects are minimized.
   c. Common cause variations are eliminated.
   d. Faulty data is removed.

15. What is the purpose of the fishbone diagram?
   a. It is designed to identify process redundancies.
   b. It is used for process evaluation.
   c. It can predict product failure.
   d. It identifies causes of an effect.

16. Which of the following choices is consistent with functional benchmarking?
   a. Preparation time of discharge medication at a hospital pharmacy vs. wait time in-person at a CVS pharmacy
   b. Hospital absentee rate for Human Resources and Dietary Services
   c. Hospital A's readmission rates compared to Hospital B's readmission rates
   d. Customer satisfaction in Hospital A and Bank of America

17. A recent pandemic has stressed the entire healthcare system. A team is evaluating the staffing needs for RN coverage. Which of the following measurements will supply the most appropriate information?
   a. Gap analysis with a fishbone diagram
   b. Agency-wide job satisfaction survey with the Employee Net promoter scale
   c. Root cause analysis with the 5 Whys
   d. Descriptive statistics on Qualtrics

18. According to the CMS Five-Star Quality Rating System, which of the following quality measures is assessed in long-term care nursing facilities but does not apply to short-term care nursing facilities?
   a. Use of restraints
   b. Presence of pressure ulcers
   c. Delirium onset
   d. Moderate to severe pain

19. Which of the following choices is consistent with the function of FMEA in healthcare systems?
   a. The process risks and system effects for actual and potential processes are identified.
   b. The measure uses the patient severity score as the basis for failure assessment.
   c. The etiology and identification of responsible parties of the process errors are explored.
   d. The reliability of the assessment is limited to potential process failures.

20. A team is charged with launching a patient portal for a large primary care network. There are 1,000 patients covered by the network. Critical mass is a quantitative measure of the eventual success of diffusion. What is the point of critical mass for the diffusion of this project?
   a. 50 patients have enrolled.
   b. 150 patients have enrolled.
   c. 300 patients have enrolled.
   d. 900 patients have enrolled.

21. The team leaders are planning a teens-only discussion group for diabetic patients. Which of the following data management systems would provide social media information related to teenage patients' needs and attitudes related to their diabetes?
   a. Individual patients' EHR records
   b. HEDIS HbA1C results
   c. Assessment of the HCRM results
   d. The result of the RCM review

22. Root cause analysis is used to identify the circumstances that led to a clinical error. Which of the following statements is consistent with a latent cause?
   a. Elevated serum glucose due to an incorrect diet order in the EHR
   b. A mechanical fall due to the administration of the wrong dose of Lisinopril
   c. An adverse reaction between two medications which was not previously identified
   d. An x-ray of the right shoulder instead of the left shoulder, which was injured

23. Belbin's team role theory identifies three descriptive categories that include action-oriented, thought-oriented, and people-oriented team characteristics. The theory then discusses three role types in each category. Which of the following team members should be the leader of the team?
   a. The people-oriented specialist
   b. The thought-oriented plant
   c. The people-oriented team worker
   d. The action-oriented shaper

24. Which of the following organizational characteristics is recognized as having the greatest effect on CMS Five-Star Quality Rating System scores?
   a. All new technologies are quickly incorporated.
   b. Senior management drives innovation.
   c. Individual departments create action plans.
   d. Continuous improvement plans drive change.

25. A SIPOC diagram identifies the Suppliers, Inputs, Process, Outputs, and Customers for a project. The team is charged with creating an eye-health program to accommodate all Medicare patients with diabetes in the health care system. Which of the following choices is a critical input for this plan?
   a. Transportation services
   b. Clinic appointment availability
   c. NP staff scheduling
   d. Patient contact

26. Based on his research in the aviation industry, James Reason applied the Swiss Cheese model of latent causation to healthcare systems. Which of the following choices is consistent with that model?
   a. Nursing staff is always involved in errors that cause actual harm.
   b. Errors occur when inherent risks in multiple system areas overlap with one another.
   c. Most of the latent causes are easily traceable and amenable to revision.
   d. The Swiss Cheese model only applies to actual errors.

27. The AHRQ is responsible for constructing and publishing the current patient safety quality indicators. Which of the following choices is a current PSI?
   a. ER admissions for mechanical falls
   b. Iatrogenic pneumothorax rate
   c. Infiltrated peripheral IV site
   d. Community-acquired sepsis

28. James Reason coined the terms *active* and *latent* causes and went on to label the active cause as the *sharp end* and the latent causes as the *blunt end* of the error. Which of the following represents the sharp end of an error?
   a. An infusion pump with a complex interface
   b. A nurse who administers the incorrect medication
   c. An outpatient center lab not connected to the system
   d. Patient portals with confusing upload instructions

29. The work breakdown structure (WBS) provides a picture of the total project that is used to evaluate team performance. Which of the following choices would NOT be included in the diagram?
   a. Deliverables
   b. Tasks
   c. Work packages
   d. Stakeholders

30. Which of the following actions would NOT be included in a HIPAA risk assessment test?
   a. Development of specific backup plans for protecting all data, including protected health information (PHI)
   b. Identification of specific rules for the storage of PHI on mobile devices
   c. Estimation of financial gains for investing in encryption technology
   d. Communication of the importance of documenting all safeguards

31. Which of the following elements is consistent with the Systems Engineering Initiative for Patient Safety (SEIPS)?
   a. Geography is one of the basic environmental factors.
   b. The people factor relates to hospitalized patients only.
   c. The theoretical framework for the plan is the medical model.
   d. The plan connects the work systems, processes, and outcomes.

32. Which of the following choices is consistent with the reporting requirements for an actual cause event?
    a. CMS notification of sentinel events is voluntary.
    b. The incident report is agency eyes-only.
    c. Adverse drug reaction reporting to the FDA is voluntary.
    d. All of the above are correct.

33. Peer evaluation is a common measure of team effectiveness. Which of the following choices is an example of reciprocity bias in peer evaluations?
    a. Carol gives everyone a 10 because she received a 10.
    b. Jack gives everyone a 10 because he thinks the whole team was successful.
    c. Fred gives everyone a 10 because he doesn't want any issues.
    d. Ann gives everyone a 5 because she isn't taking the blame for poor team performance.

34. Which of the following choices is true about Medicaid eligibility as defined by the Affordable Care Act?
    a. Individual states were required to adopt the new rules.
    b. The Supreme Court ruled that states could choose to expand coverage.
    c. The new rules addressed eligibility for children and adults.
    d. All fifty states have experienced increased adult and child enrollment.

35. A modified SWOT framework can be used as a performance evaluation measure by substituting the identification of "areas for improvement" for "weaknesses." How does this framework benefit the employee?
    a. The employee can challenge the evaluation criteria.
    b. The employee can set the record straight about any adverse comments.
    c. The employee can identify additional resources that would be beneficial.
    d. The employee can report team members who are not meeting team goals.

36. Which of the following is consistent with the current focus of the Core Quality Measures Collaborative (CQMC)?
    a. Address disparity of care issues associated with the existing core measures.
    b. Issue post-pandemic recommendations for the use of personal protective equipment (PPE).
    c. Update core measures that relate to antibiotic management for infectious diseases.
    d. Establish recommendations for emergency management of opioid overdoses.

37. Which of the following choices is consistent with systems thinking for risk reduction in a healthcare system?
    a. The identification of connections among different departments is required.
    b. The resulting plan is applicable to all patient-care units.
    c. Systems thinking only applies to high-risk areas such as nursing.
    d. Smaller healthcare systems do not benefit from systems thinking.

38. A team in a large primary care system is creating a plan to meet the CMS (Medicare) requirement for scheduling annual wellness visits for all patients covered by Medicare. Which of the following choices is consistent with a process failure for this project?
   a. Eighteen percent of the eligible members scheduled an appointment.
   b. The patient portal was used to announce the program.
   c. The area received 10 inches of rain.
   d. The system server was down for 3 days during the enrollment period.

39. Which of the following choices is consistent with the primary focus of the Institute for Comparative Clinical Effectiveness Research?
   a. Improved treatment options for specific diseases
   b. Research protocols that use only quantitative designs
   c. Population-health interventions
   d. Financial support for large research projects

40. Which of the following choices is NOT an assessment domain included in the HEDIS database?
   a. Care effectiveness
   b. Care access and availability
   c. Cumulative costs of care
   d. EHR data capture and reporting

41. Which of the following certification criteria was added in the restructuring of the Magnet plan in 2008?
   a. Transformational leadership
   b. Exemplary professional practice
   c. Outcomes reporting
   d. Generation of new knowledge

42. When applied to project planning, what does the quote "significant few - trivial many" refer to?
   a. It means that 80 percent of the variance is due to 20 percent of the causes.
   b. It refers to an environmental cause result of FMEA analysis.
   c. It is the KPI comparison of average hospital stay and bed turnover.
   d. It is an alternate expression of the fishbone diagram.

43. The annual Medicare Health Outcomes Survey uses the HEDIS database information to evaluate patient care. Who completes the survey?
   a. All patients over sixty-five years old who receive Medicare benefits
   b. Randomly selected Medicare patients
   c. Providers who care for patients over sixty-five years old
   d. Hospitals that admit Medicare patients

44. Which of the following statements is consistent with thought mapping?
   a. The thought map is created by the Six Sigma process champion.
   b. The quality of the final thought map depends on strict adherence to the construction process.
   c. The thought map should be created prior to addressing the DMAIC questions.
   d. The thought map identifies the questions that will be prioritized in the DMAIC process.

45. Which of the following industry certifications is based on outcome measures of clinical performance and consumer satisfaction?
   a. Joint Commission on Accreditation of Healthcare Organizations (JCAHO)
   b. National Committee for Quality Assurance (NCQA)
   c. Utilization Review Accreditation Commission (URAC)
   d. American Association for Ambulatory Health Care (AAAHC)

46. Human factors engineering addresses the complex relationships between humans and healthcare technology. Which of the following choices is consistent with a work-around?
   a. An alternative process that decreases risk
   b. A time-saving short-cut
   c. A process that bypasses safeguards
   d. A detailed analysis of the steps of a process

47. What is the function of validation concerning the process improvement protocol?
   a. Validation ensures that the identified solutions are appropriate to the project outcomes.
   b. Validation identifies gaps in the "knowns."
   c. Validation confirms that the completed outcome solves the problem.
   d. Validation suggests the appropriate choice of Six Sigma tools.

48. The Best-Care Hospital team leaders are evaluating the effectiveness of the Ambulatory Surgical Care unit that was opened last year. Which of the following classifications of data analytical procedures provide specific recommendations for implementing new innovations based on past performance?
   a. Prescriptive analytics
   b. Predictive analytics
   c. Descriptive analytics
   d. Diagnostic analytics

49. The International Standards Organization (ISO) sets standards for multiple disciplines and activities that are used as quality benchmarks worldwide. Which of the following choices is consistent with the ISO certification process?
   a. ISO certification is required for CMS reimbursement.
   b. ISO standards supersede competing standards from other agencies.
   c. ISO agency certification must be renewed every five years.
   d. ISO certification requires an independent audit of agency compliance.

50. One result of human factors engineering is the addition of the forced function limitation aimed at decreasing the human factor associated with a process. Which of the following is an example of this safeguard?
   a. The medication is delivered in unit-dose amounts.
   b. A signature is required to obtain controlled substances.
   c. Computer provider order entry (CPOE) is required for EHR orders.
   d. Vials of potassium chloride (KCl) are removed from nursing units.

51. When assessing the progress of a performance improvement project, what is the most discrete form of a deliverable that can be evaluated?

a. Work package
b. Project outcomes
c. KPIs
d. Project scope

52. The Baldrige Award for organizational excellence evaluates every aspect of the organizational structure. Hospital leaders are cautioned to address the effects of disruptive technology, such as social media, precision management models, and artificial intelligence (AI) innovations on organizational performance. What is the most critical consequence of failing to plan for disruptive technology?

a. Negative effects on the competitive environment
b. Increased costs of technology implementation
c. Possible HIPAA penalties
d. Staffing deficiencies

53. Which of the following statements is consistent with the current CMS AI systems reimbursement plan for providers?

a. CMS does not reimburse AI systems.
b. All radiology procedures now use AI for final diagnoses.
c. AI costs are transferred to the individual patient.
d. CMS reimburses for FDA pre-certified AI systems.

54. Which of the following choices is NOT a characteristic of risk management in a high-reliability healthcare system?

a. Relies on retrospective error assessment
b. Views untoward events as opportunities for improvement
c. Sees the entire workforce as responsible for risk reduction
d. Maintains transparency of risk reduction activities

55. According to Six Sigma methodology, when is the appropriate point in a process improvement project to conduct a cost-benefit analysis?

a. At the start of the project charter
b. During the define stage
c. At intervals throughout the implementation
d. The assessment is required at each of these points.

56. The Commission on Accreditation of Rehabilitation Facilities (CARF) is an international non-profit organization that sets standards and provides accreditation for a wide range of ambulatory care services. Which of the following choices is true about CARF?

a. The commission is federally funded.
b. Third-party payers require accreditation of individual facilities.
c. Consumers can identify accredited care facilities.
d. Accreditation is limited to adult-care facilities.

57. The team is assessing the launch of a new watch that has several applications not available in any other watch. Which of the following choices is consistent with the definitions of innovators and early adopters in the Diffusion of Innovation model?
    a. Innovators need to possess the first edition model of the watch.
    b. Early adopters wait to see if the watch works as advertised.
    c. Innovators base their decisions on price of the watch.
    d. Early adopters will buy the watch after reading about the technology.

58. The Fast Healthcare Interoperability Resource (FHIR) standards are used to optimize the applications for improving data interoperability in healthcare. Which of the following might be a patient experience outcome resulting from this technology?
    a. Comparison of national and regional HbA1C level trends
    b. Elimination of multiple patient portals
    c. Early identification of diabetic neuropathy
    d. Point-of-care documentation of providers' costs

59. The team leaders of the newly opened Best-Care Hospital are deciding which accreditations would be most useful to the function of the new community hospital. Which of the following accreditations should be the highest priority for this team?
    a. Magnet
    b. Joint Commission on Accreditation of Healthcare Organizations (JCAHO)
    c. International Standards Organization (ISO)
    d. Baldridge Award

60. According to the Joint Commission rules, who is responsible for marking the surgical site pre-operatively?
    a. The provider - most commonly the surgeon
    b. Certified Nurse Practitioner
    c. Licensed Physician's Assistant
    d. All of the above

61. At what point in the DMAIC model would a value stream map be used?
    a. Define
    b. Measure
    c. Analyze
    d. Improve

62. What is the purpose of Quality Core Measures?
    a. To coordinate care metrics only for private payers
    b. To simplify fee-for-service documentation
    c. To focus on care quality, not costs
    d. To facilitate implementation of value-based care

63. Which of the following choices is consistent with the JCAHO Survey Analysis for Evaluating Risk Matrix that addresses the Requirement for Improvement (RFI) noncompliance items?
   a. The matrix categorizes each RFI according to patient risk.
   b. Agency improvements must be documented within six months of the JCAHO visit.
   c. The matrix score is based on the number of times the error was made.
   d. All RFIs will be investigated in subsequent JCAHO onsite reviews.

64. Six Sigma would be the most effective management system for which of the following entities?
   a. Children's Art School
   b. The Widget Company
   c. Best-Care Health System
   d. AI Software Team

65. Which of the following infection control issues has been identified as a priority in the NPSG (National Patient Safety Goals) 2022 initiative by the Joint Commission and WHO?
   a. PPE (personal protective equipment) use
   b. IV site dressing technique
   c. Handwashing
   d. Environmental infection controls

66. The Occupational Health and Safety Administration (OSHA) sets standards for employee safety in the workplace. Which of the following areas is NOT addressed by OSHA standards?
   a. Workplace violence
   b. Patient transfer ergonomics
   c. Potential for infectious contamination
   d. Workers' Compensation claims

67. Which of the following steps of mistake proofing is used most frequently?
   a. Facilitation
   b. Elimination
   c. Replacement
   d. Mitigation

68. Which of the following choices is consistent with the Consumers Assessment of Healthcare Providers and Systems survey (CAHPS)?
   a. Healthcare researchers pay a nominal fee for access to the data.
   b. The purpose of the survey is to assess patients' experience with the healthcare system.
   c. CMS requires all providers to collect the CAHPS data every two years to survey CMS patients.
   d. The survey is only appropriate for the evaluation of primary care providers.

69. The PIP (Performance Improvement Plan) documents the performance of individual team members. The plan commonly uses numerical ratings to quantify performance. These systems are not favored by either managers or team members. A three-part evaluation system that addresses growth, plans for improvement, and support (called GPS) has been proposed. How would this plan benefit the manager?
   a. The plan wouldn't benefit the manager because the numerical system is more objective.
   b. It would be easier to impose consequences of continued sub-standard performance.
   c. The manager could identify company resources that would improve individual performance.
   d. The plan would decrease the number of merit raises with better performance assessment.

70. Which of the following KPIs is specifically identified as a healthcare financial metric?
   a. Bed or room turnover
   b. Processing time for insurance claims
   c. Average patient wait time in radiology
   d. Medical equipment utilization

71. Which of the following choices is consistent with internal and competitive benchmarking by team leaders?
   a. It is a cost-effective way to improve care outcomes.
   b. Benchmarking is the most important element of process change.
   c. Innovation is stimulated when hospitals meet benchmarks.
   d. The results of benchmarking data types are interchangeable.

72. Which of the following choices is NOT considered to be a benefit of a cost-benefit analysis?
   a. It is based on objective assessment data.
   b. The completed plan provides a decision-making framework.
   c. It removes the human element from decisions.
   d. The construction of the plan offers new insights.

73. When the Lean Six Sigma methodology is used in a healthcare system, what is the primary outcome?
   a. Improves financial position
   b. Decreases use of temporary staffing
   c. Controls inherent patient risk
   d. Increases market share

74. The COVID-19 pandemic identified gaps in the United States healthcare system's response to a novel infectious agent. In response to these deficiencies, the National Emerging Special Pathogens Training and Education Center (NETEC) developed the National Special Pathogen System of Care (NSPS) model. Which of the following choices is consistent with that model?
   a. The implementation of the model is funded by private individuals.
   b. Participation in the plan is voluntary.
   c. All care facilities will implement the complete model.
   d. A Central Body will coordinate implementation of the model.

75. The team is evaluating the rate of innovation diffusion for their latest project. The adoption behavior of which of the following individuals is the best predictor of the success of the innovation?
   a. The laggards because if they're convinced, the process must be successful.
   b. The late majority because this group is skeptical but will go with the majority.
   c. The early majority because they will implement the innovation before the average person.
   d. The early adopter because they implement earlier, and they are perceived as leaders.

76. The Lean Six Sigma methodology focuses on seven areas of waste in the system. What is the eighth waste that typically results from the previous wastes?
   a. Human potential
   b. Excess motion
   c. Over-processing
   d. Wait times

77. Which of the following choices is true about potential barriers to the use of machine learning in healthcare settings?
   a. Free-form narrative EHR data is not intelligible.
   b. The process is too expensive for individual providers.
   c. It doesn't decrease human input time.
   d. Machine learning doesn't improve reimbursement.

78. Which of the following is consistent with the goals of the NSPS model?
   a. Mobilization of the care network with 24 hours of threat identification
   b. Greater than 95% community accessibility to care
   c. Zero preventable deaths among patients infected with special pathogens
   d. 100% patient satisfaction with the level of care

79. A team is preparing the final Six Sigma report for a process improvement project that examined the production of an improved charging system for a cardiac pacemaker. The team adds the GR&R report to the measure documentation section of the report. Which of the following choices is consistent with the purpose of the GR&R report?
   a. Calculation of process variation
   b. Estimation of stakeholder satisfaction
   c. Calculation of root cause analysis
   d. Determination of sample size

80. The Lean Six Sigma methodology uses the 5S process that was adapted from the Toyota model to address workplace organization. Which of the following choices is consistent with the *standardize* step of the process?
   a. Environmental cleanliness
   b. Color-coded patient care items
   c. Clutter-free environment
   d. Standardized inventory for Level 2 nursing units

81. Which of the following choices is consistent with the agency impact of a negative CMS or OSHA review?
   a. Liability insurance costs may be increased.
   b. Errors that are corrected within sixty days are not published.
   c. Patient information resources do not include error reporting for hospitals.
   d. Individual performance evaluation is non-punitive.

82. The IHI recommends the use of specific measures to track Triple Aim solution efforts. Which of the following assessments addresses the health of the population?
   a. ED utilization rate
   b. The Institute of Medicine (IOM) Quality Chasm Assessment
   c. Composite Health Risk Appraisal (HRA) score
   d. Consumer Assessment of Provider and Systems global measures

83. Which of the following statements is consistent with the anticipated results of the implementation of the Six Sigma methodology for process and product quality improvement?
    a. Company revenue increases.
    b. The product price increases.
    c. Time spent on future QI decreases.
    d. Employee satisfaction decreases.

84. Team leaders in the Best-Care Hospital have successfully implemented a major innovation in direct patient care. What is the next step of the process?
    a. Develop performance evaluation measures.
    b. Identify a sustainability model for the changes.
    c. Publish the success of the innovations.
    d. Apply the implementation process to the next problem.

85. A team is reviewing the concept of value-added and non-value-added activities. Which of the following activities is a customer value-added activity?
    a. Decreased product transit time
    b. Workstation redesign
    c. Digitization of inventory control
    d. Employee skills evaluation

86. Which of the following is an example of a "never event"?
    a. Surgical instrument left in the operative site
    b. Wound infection
    c. Grade 4 pressure ulcer
    d. IV site phlebitis

87. Four newly licensed physicians are planning to open a group practice to provide a broad range of eye-care services. According to Porter's Five Forces of Competition, how will the threat of new entrants affect their practice?
    a. Advancing technologies limit competition.
    b. Medical tourism has expanded the competitive market.
    c. Existing patient-provider relationships constrain competition.
    d. All of the above are correct.

88. Which of the following choices is NOT consistent with the use of a balanced scorecard?
    a. Future technology needs are identified.
    b. The connections between key objectives are more visible.
    c. The strategic plan is visible to all employees.
    d. The scorecard works best for small businesses.

89. The NCQA has developed the Quality Compass, which is a proprietary software program. Which of the following choices is consistent with this measure?
    a. The results of competitive benchmarking are provided.
    b. The measure produces a checklist for reporting deadlines.
    c. HEDIS and CAHPS consumer data is analyzed.
    d. The program submits prepared data directly to CMS.

90. Which of the following choices is consistent with the concept of team cohesiveness?
   a. All team members agree with one another.
   b. The team is committed to the success of the project.
   c. Cohesiveness is created by the leader.
   d. Team cohesion develops in Tuckman's norming stage.

91. Which of the following choices identifies the difference between the FMEA level 2 outcome severity rating and the FMEA level 3 outcome severity rating?
   a. Level 3 occurrences are reportable in most states.
   b. Level 2 occurrences require additional patient care services.
   c. Level 3 occurrences could prompt process revision.
   d. Level 2 occurrences are largely preventable.

92. America's Health Insurance Plans (AHIP) publishes core measures of excellence across nine specialties. Which of the following choices is consistent with this program?
   a. The core measures are specific to value-based payment programs.
   b. All care outcomes are measured by consumer self-report surveys.
   c. The core measure reports are required by CMS.
   d. The core measures are only applicable to acute-care settings.

93. Which of the following choices is consistent with the purpose of the Accrediting Council for Continuing Medical Education (ACME)?
   a. Provide CMS-compliant accreditation for individual providers
   b. Monitor providers' completion of required continuing education credit hours
   c. Set standards for continuing medical education credit offerings
   d. Document program completion for pre-licensure students

94. According to the theory of Diffusion of Information, at what point in the process does the person assess the utility of the new idea?
   a. Persuasion
   b. Decision
   c. Implementation
   d. Confirmation

95. Which of the following choices is consistent with the uses of Enterprise Management Software (EMS) programs?
   a. Develop preventive maintenance schedules for HVAC systems.
   b. Coordinate Human Resources management.
   c. Capture patient satisfaction data.
   d. Consolidate patients' medical records.

96. The AHRQ has published quality indicators for inpatient conditions such as pressure ulcers, central line infections, and postoperative sepsis. Which of the following choices is the primary focus of the indicators?
   a. Improved patient satisfaction
   b. Identification of prevention strategies
   c. Accurate CMS reimbursement
   d. Implementation of performance evaluation plans

97. The team is developing a process map for the launch of a new and improved widget. Which of the following choices is NOT included in the process map for the scope of the QI project?
   a. Identification of raw materials and information resources
   b. List of the widget production steps from start to finish
   c. Description of the new and improved widget
   d. Distribution of the new widget to loyal customers

98. Which of the following choices is consistent with CMS bundled payment?
   a. Providers assume additional financial risk.
   b. Medical patient-care bundles have lowered costs.
   c. CMS captures all financial losses when targets are not met.
   d. Surgical patient transfer to skilled nursing facilities decreases costs.

99. There are three terms used in the Six Sigma method that describe waste as defined by the Toyota model: *muda*, *mura*, and *muri*. *Muda* is often used to describe the entire model; however, the three terms do have distinct definitions. *Muda* refers to the seven classic waste categories of Six Sigma. *Mura* describes circumstances where there is inconsistent production due to one of the seven wastes. *Muri* refers to excessive stress on the worker, which also often results from one of the seven wastes. Which of the following choices would be consistent with *muri*?
   a. The first quarter report revealed significant week-to-week variation in production.
   b. The average production time rose twelve percent per unit last month.
   c. The individual average weekly total was fifty-six hours per week last month.
   d. Repeat customers provided negative feedback for the new modifications of the product.

100. Which of the following choices is consistent with the Sentinel Event Measure of Success (SEMOS) measure?
   a. It is a reporting tool for a sentinel evident occurrence.
   b. It is an evaluation measure of the sentinel action plan.
   c. It is the comparison between sentinel events and near misses.
   d. It categorizes the root causes of the sentinel events.

101. The nursing staff are investigating a recent increase in central line infections. Which of the following charts would be most useful?
   a. Run chart
   b. Histogram
   c. Fishbone
   d. Pareto chart

102. Which of the following choices is consistent with a Pareto chart?
   a. The 80/20 rule for causation always applies.
   b. There are multiple ways to express the data.
   c. The results will identify areas for improvement.
   d. Root cause analysis of the useful many is identified.

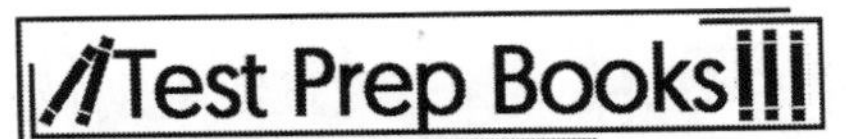

103. The team is trying to identify characteristics of the variation in a new process. Which of the following instruments will provide the best answers?
   a. Pareto chart
   b. Statistical Process Control (SPC) chart
   c. FMEA chart
   d. Fishbone diagram

104. Which of the following choices is consistent with the RC squared ($RCA^2$ ) analysis?
   a. FMEA results are more reliable.
   b. SBAR produces the same results in less time.
   c. The Joint Commission doesn't recognize the resulting data.
   d. The analysis requires the development and review of an action plan.

105. Which of the following choices is consistent with competitive benchmarking in healthcare?
   a. Hospital bed capacity is the most critical KPI.
   b. Climate conditions can affect hospital comparisons.
   c. Hospital metrics in the same geographic locations are comparable.
   d. Measurement of KPIs is not affected by demographic differences.

106. Which of the following choices is consistent with generic benchmarking?
   a. Comparison of similar processes in similar organizations
   b. Comparison of the same process in individual departments in an organization
   c. Comparison of similar processes in dissimilar organizations
   d. Comparison of similar concepts in disparate organizations

107. Six Sigma methodology is commonly represented as $Y = f(x)$. Which of the following statements is consistent with this formula?
   a. The equation is specific to the Six Sigma process improvement model.
   b. The equation is used only in the "D" or "define" step of the DMAIC model.
   c. The equation is limited to the identification of process errors.
   d. The equation defines all aspects of process evaluation.

108. Which of the following choices is consistent with the Hospital Consumer Assessment of Healthcare Providers and Systems (HCAHPS) survey?
   a. Pain satisfaction results are highly correlated with postoperative opioid therapy.
   b. Higher overall patient satisfaction scores are associated with positive clinical outcomes.
   c. The survey results do not affect CMS payments in states that administer Medicaid.
   d. There are concerns about the validity of patient satisfaction as a reimbursement metric.

109. Which of the following instruments would be the best indicator for the success of Six Sigma process improvement?
   a. The measurement of ROI
   b. Determination of cause and effect
   c. Calculation of the failure potential
   d. Identification of pilot test results

110. Which of the following choices is a possible effect of groupthink on the brainstorming phase of quality improvement planning?
   a. Everyone expresses the same idea.
   b. Group ideas are unrealistic.
   c. Group engagement is limited.
   d. Each group is self-reliant.

111. During which stage of the Know What, Know How, Know Why improvement huddle model are the key points discussed?
   a. Know What
   b. Know How
   c. Know Why
   d. Introduction

112. What is the primary function of Tuckman's forming stage?
   a. Reflecting on group process
   b. Resolving team differences
   c. Identifying individual competence
   d. Encouraging team communication

113. The Science of Improvement identifies three types of healthcare improvement measures. Which of the following choices exemplifies a balancing measure?
   a. Use of ventilator bundle versus re-intubation rates
   b. Semi-annual HbA1c testing for diabetic patients
   c. Adverse drug reactions per quarter
   d. Completion of on-time intentional rounding

114. Which of the following conditions would be addressed in the *analyze* step of the DMAIC model in a healthcare system?
   a. Fifty percent of eligible clinic patients received a flu shot before October 31.
   b. One hundred percent of eligible clinic patients will receive a flu shot before October 31.
   c. An immunization tracking process is implemented.
   d. The tracking protocol is applied to a patient-portal engagement initiative.

115. Which of the following choices distinguishes between the Merit-Based Incentive Payment System (MIPS) and the Advanced Alternative Payment Model (APM) CMS reimbursement plans?
   a. Verification of EHR usage is not required for APM organizations.
   b. APM organizations assume additional financial risk.
   c. MIPS organizations receive greater financial incentives.
   d. Smaller provider groups are not currently eligible for either program.

116. The AHRQ developed the SHARE model (Seek, Help, Assess, Reach, Evaluate) to facilitate patients' involvement in making healthcare decisions. Which of the following choices is the focus of the Assess step of the model?
   a. Rehabilitation potential
   b. Clinical pathway progress
   c. Patient's personal values
   d. DRG for admitting diagnosis

117. Which of the following individuals would most commonly be responsible for identifying potential team members?
    a. Direct manager
    b. Peer member
    c. Senior manager
    d. Employee

118. Which of the following choices is NOT an expected outcome of the SHARE model?
    a. Positive patient compliance with the treatment plan
    b. Increased cost of care savings
    c. Improved care outcomes
    d. Better patient-care experiences

119. Artificial Intelligence (AI) innovations are increasingly being used to harness the potential of EHR patient data. Which of the following areas is the target for the AI natural language processing (NLP) model?
    a. Predictive analytics
    b. Clinical documentation
    c. Care decision algorithms
    d. Diagnostic radiology

120. What does force field analysis measure in the Six Sigma model?
    a. Error percentage per unit
    b. Process time management
    c. Inventory controls
    d. Plus and minus factors

121. Which of the following information sources is provided by patients for patients?
    a. Healthcare Effectiveness Data and Information Set (HEDIS) databases
    b. Core Quality Measures reports
    c. America's Health Insurance Plans (AHIP) reports
    d. Consumer Assessment of Healthcare Providers and Systems (CAHPS) data

122. The availability of new biosimilar and generic drugs is projected to lower drug costs. Which of the following choices identifies a barrier to savings for Medicare patients related to the use of biosimilar drugs?
    a. There are no biosimilar drugs used for hypertension.
    b. Patients are reluctant to use these new drug forms.
    c. Many biosimilar drugs lack interchangeability.
    d. Biosimilar drugs are not covered in all Part D drug plan formularies

123. What is the main purpose of work packages in the project scope management process?
    a. They establish the price per unit.
    b. They provide attainable project work units.
    c. They track inventory control.
    d. They identify performance evaluation points.

124. Which of the following choices is consistent with the CMS Hospital Value-Based Purchasing Program?
   a. Incentives are limited to conditions with high readmission rates.
   b. Incentive payments are related to quality outcomes.
   c. The clinical outcomes score is the single payment metric.
   d. Ambulatory surgical centers are included in the program.

125. Which of the following choices is consistent with the focus of structured terminologies?
   a. Design of hardware configurations
   b. Conversion of EHR narrative documentation
   c. Elimination of unauthorized data access
   d. Decrease in immediate staff learning needs

# Answer Explanations #3

**1. A:** The strategy is focused on transforming attitudes, behavior, and practice by encouraging consideration of four values: accountability, health literacy, respect, and patient-centered care. This means that Choice *A* is correct, and the remaining choices are incorrect.

**2. A:** The mode is the most frequently appearing number in the sequence. Choice *A* is also the median for this group of results, which is the number in the middle when the results are arranged in numerical order. Choice *B* is the mean (average) of the results. Choices *C* and *D* are incorrect as well; they are the highest and lowest point in the data set, respectively.

**3. C:** The correct answer is Choice *C* because, by definition, the consulted person is a team member who provides input but is not directly responsible for doing the work. Choice *A* is incorrect because the responsible person does the work. There should be only one responsible person for the project, and that person would be an employee rather than a manager. The accountable person is a manager who is responsible for approving the completed work, so Choice *B* is incorrect. The informed person is made aware of the progress of the project but does not contribute to the work; therefore, Choice *D* is incorrect.

**4. C:** Organizations must design patient information resources that are accessible and easily understandable to improve patient engagement in the healthcare process. Discharge information should be patient-specific with clear instructions for supporting or additional information sources. Contact alternatives for patient portals must also be available. Aside from the obvious consideration for alternative language, the resources must also consider reading literacy levels. The remaining choices are potential organizational benefits; however, increased patient engagement is beneficial for patients and organizations. This means that Choices *A, B,* and *D* are incorrect.

**5. D:** Leaders are cautioned that team members can become frustrated with the preliminary work that must be completed at the outset of the forming stage; therefore, Choice *D* is correct. Team members in the storming stage can become competitive as everyone begins to be more open by sharing their ideas and opinions. This means that Choice *A* is incorrect. In the norming stage, the team becomes a cohesive entity that agrees with the plan going forward; therefore, Choice *B* is incorrect. The team members function autonomously in the performing stage and are strongly motivated to see the successful outcomes of their work, which means that Choice *C* is incorrect.

**6. D:** Statistical process control (SPC) measures identify variations in time-series process data. Common cause variations are inherent in the process, and special cause variations are process effects that occur spontaneously and may or may not be repeated over time. Common cause variations require attention to the process and are often identified as areas for quality improvement assessment. Special cause variations prompt attention to the cause of the variation rather than the process. For instance, two patients are waiting for an appointment at the pain clinic. They each experience a ten-day wait; however, patient A waited ten days because the EHR did not transmit the request from the PCP to the clinic.

Patient B waited ten days because one of the pain clinic specialists was on vacation and the other specialist broke her leg last week. To improve patient A's experience, the system requires attention because the referral process is an expected function of the EHR. The solution for patient B could be to increase the number of specialists in the pain clinic (i.e., address the cause of the wait time). Choice *A* is incorrect because the process variations identified by SPC measures dictate the details of the quality improvement efforts. The results of the SPC analysis can track improvement in a process over time, but there is no statistical "proof" that the quality improvement measures were responsible for the improvement, which means that Choice *B* is incorrect. SPC measures are used to identify common cause variations and special cause variations, which means that Choice *C* is incorrect.

**7. B:** The organization is responsible for providing both current technology resources and readily available support associated with the use of the technology. Under "normal" circumstances, the remaining choices would not be directly controlled by the leaders of the organization, which means that Choices *A, C,* and *D* are incorrect.

**8. B**: If the leader is unable to manage the inevitable conflict of the storming stage, the entire project may be affected. The work of the other phases may be affected; however, the changes in group dynamics during the storming stage present the greatest challenge to the team leader. Therefore, Choice *B* is correct.

**9. C:** Trend analysis is a visual representation of the changes in a process over time; however, team leaders are reminded that the SPC measures do not automatically provide the analysis of the observed trends. The trends are described as general, linear, nonlinear, or systematic, and the trend patterns do not repeat during the observed interval. Trend analysis is not produced by SPC measures, which means that Choice *A* is incorrect. The trend pattern does not repeat in the observed time frame, so Choice *B* is incorrect. Trend patterns may be negative or positive linear figures or random systematic patterns, which means that Choice *D* is incorrect.

**10. B:** A sentinel event is an error committed by an individual that results in harm or death of one or more persons, which means that Choice *B* is the correct answer. Choice *A* is incorrect because the designation of an error as sentinel has no relationship with the time interval between the commission of the error and the reporting of the error. Choice *C* is incorrect because sentinel events result in harm to the patient because of an action committed by another individual. The precipitating cause may be organizational; however, the sentinel event is an individual act. Choice *D* is the definition of a near-miss event, which means that Choice *D* is incorrect.

**11. D:** The electronic transmission of prescriptions is one of the activities included in phase 3 of the Meaningful Use Initiative. In general, the phase 3 requirements address individual patient outcomes and levels of engagement. This is in contrast to the first two phases, which address public health issues. Additional requirements for phase 3 include clinical quality measures reporting, patient interaction via the patient portal, and Computerized Provider Order Entry. Providers are required to meet one of the public health issues identified in Choices *A, B,* and *C*, and phase 2 requires additional reporting for each of these measures. This means that Choices *A, B,* and *C* are incorrect.

**12. B:** Choice *B* identifies a threat to patient safety because the numbers that are entered control the infusion, and there is potential for error if the lighting for the front of the prototype is poorly designed. This would receive the highest score for severity among the four choices because the defect occurs frequently in patient-care areas, and the defect is immediately obvious to the customer. An extension that is difficult to attach would be a problem of moderate severity; the defect could potentially occur every time the infusion was used, and the defect would be obvious to the customer.

However, this problem is less of a threat to patient safety because the extension cord does fit the infusion pump with some effort. This means that Choice *A* is incorrect. Device alarms are also connected to patient safety; however, in this instance, the alarm is functioning, but the volume cannot be regulated. This issue would also occur with every use of the pump and would be obvious; however, this defect is less severe than the control panel issue, so Choice *C* is incorrect. The only concern associated with the weight of the machine is the quality of the system that attaches the pump to the IV pole, so the severity is less of a threat to patient safety. Based on the severity alone, Choice *D* is incorrect.

**13. B:** The rating system was developed in response to the escalating costs for hospital readmission within thirty days of discharge. Many of these readmissions were related to poor communication in the transition of care. The Five-Star Rating System requires documentation of the following: notification of the primary provider of the patient's admission and discharge, and face-to-face patient engagement and medication reconciliation by the primary provider within 30 days of discharge. Choices *A, C,* and *D* are incorrect because their measures are included in the Five-Star Quality Rating System.

**14. B:** Using the median value to smooth data statistically decreases the effects of the outliers to a greater degree than using the mean value. There are currently no automatic ways to identify data trends. They are identified by visual assessment of the SPC output, which means that Choice *A* is incorrect. Common cause variations cannot be eliminated because they are inherent to the process, which means that Choice *C* is incorrect. Faulty data is removed in the data scrubbing process before the analysis phase, which means that Choice *D* is incorrect.

**15. D:** The fishbone diagram provides a structure for the identification of all causes related to one effect. The team brainstorms all possible influences on the effect and then uses the fishbone structure to categorize the causes. Choices *A* and *B* are incorrect because the fishbone diagram is concerned with cause and effect rather than process. Choice *C* is incorrect because the fishbone diagram does not predict product failure.

**16. A:** Functional benchmarking is defined as the comparison of related processes in dissimilar industries. The similar process is the preparation of the patients' medications, and the dissimilar industries are the hospital and the retail drugstore. Internal benchmarking compares the identical metric in different groups within the hospital, which is what Choice *B* describes—measuring absenteeism in two different departments. Choice *C* is an example of competitor benchmarking, which is defined as the measurement of a common metric (hospital readmission rates) between two hospitals. This means that Choice *C* is incorrect. Choice *D* is an example of generic benchmarking, which compares a similar metric—customer satisfaction—between two unrelated groups, Hospital A and the Bank of America. This means that Choice *D* is incorrect.

**17. A:** Gap analysis measures the difference between where an institution is with an issue (such as RN staffing) and where it needs to be. The fishbone diagram is an appropriate framework for that metric, which means that Choice *A* is correct. Measurement of RN job satisfaction would provide information about the nurses' satisfaction with organizational support during the pandemic; however, the team is trying to identify the appropriate staffing levels according to an objective measurement. This means that Choice *B* is incorrect. Root cause analysis determines the cause for an effect. In this scenario, the cause of the variances in the staffing levels is not the question; therefore, Choice *C* is incorrect. Descriptive statistics do not answer the question, which means that Choice *D* is incorrect as well.

**18. A:** The use of restraints is a quality measure for long-term settings, but not short-term settings. The remaining issues are assessed for both care settings, meaning that Choices *B, C,* and *D* are incorrect.

**19. A:** The FMEA (failure mode and effect analysis) measures the gravity of the patient effects, the potential frequency of the failure, and the likelihood that the patient will recognize the effects of actual and potential system failures. This means that Choice *A* is correct because it addresses the process, how often the failure may occur, and the patient effects. Choice *B* is incorrect because the patient severity score is only one dimension of the FMEA. Choice *C* is incorrect because the FMEA measure is focused on the prevention of system errors rather than causation. The FMEA is used to assess both actual and potential system failures, which means that Choice *D* is incorrect.

**20. B**: In this example, the critical mass for diffusion theory says that when ten to twenty percent of a population enrolls in the portal, diffusion will succeed. That means that Choice *B* is correct. Choice *A* is incorrect because it is below the critical mass. Choices *C* and *D* are incorrect because they exceed the minimum point of critical mass.

**21. C:** The HCRM measure integrates information from multiple sources, including social media. The team leaders can search this information to identify successful strategies for their new program. The EHR records and the HEDIS data would provide useful clinical information for the team; however, these databases are not integrated with social media sources, which means that Choices *A* and *B* are incorrect. RCM evaluates equipment maintenance risks that would not provide useful information for the team. So, Choice *D* is incorrect.

**22. C:** A latent cause is defined as a system error that led to an actual error, most often a human error. For instance, the actual cause is that the nurse administered the medications after reviewing the patient's pharmacy profile and available printed resources. The latent cause is that the medications are new to the market and the manufacturer's RCA measures have not yet identified the type of reaction that occurred. This means that Choice *C* is correct. Choice *A* is incorrect because the human error of incorrect order entry in the EHR was the actual cause of the elevated blood glucose. Choice *B* is incorrect because the actual cause of patient harm was due to the nurse's administration of an incorrect dose of the antihypertensive medication. Choice *D* is incorrect because the actual cause, the technician's error was the source of the potential harm to the patient due to unnecessary radiation exposure.

**23. D:** According to Belbin's theory, the action-oriented shaper takes the lead in a team situation and can problem solve and manage the team. That means that Choice *D* is correct. Choice *A* is incorrect because the people-oriented specialist focuses on specific details of the project rather than the whole project. Choice *B* is incorrect because the thought-oriented plant is a creative person who excels in the design process, not the management of the overall process. The people-oriented team worker focuses on taking care of the team members and managing conflicts that arise rather than coordinating the entire project. Therefore, Choice *C* is incorrect.

**24. D:** Healthcare organizations that achieve the highest scores have comprehensive continuous improvement plans that allow them to respond effectively to changes, maintain excellent patient care, and attract and retain exceptional employees. The most successful plans involve all stakeholders, including senior management, employees, and members of the community. Technology costs money, which means that a purposeful appraisal of the costs and benefits of new technologies would be more appropriate than implementing them immediately. This means that Choice *A* is incorrect; successful institutions would employ a more thorough approach to the incorporation of new technology. The extent to which members at all levels are involved in quality improvement efforts is one of the key indicators of organizational success. This means that Choice *B* is incorrect; proposals for change in top-down models are generally less well-received by employees. Choice *C* is incorrect because the model could result in competing plans that do not solve an organizational problem. Individual departments would be responsible for addressing issues that are specific to their work; however, successful plans for the entire organization must incorporate a holistic view.

**25. B:** According to the SIPOC diagram, the availability of clinic appointments is a critical input because the program cannot proceed if patients are not able to schedule time for the eye exam. The transportation services and NP staff are considered suppliers in the SIPOC diagram because they bring required resources to the project; therefore, Choices *A* and *C* are incorrect. Choice *D* is incorrect because patient contact is a required process for the project.

**26. B:** The Swiss Cheese model of latent causation views every area of the system as a piece of cheese with holes that represent potential areas of risk. When the holes of two or more areas overlap with one another, an error occurs. In this view, there will always be more than one source of latent causation for any actual cause. This means that Choice *B* is correct. Choice *A* is incorrect because there are multiple latent sources of actual patient harm in every healthcare system. Choice *C* is also incorrect because latent means are not easily identifiable, and successful root cause analysis depends on the resolution of those issues. The Swiss Cheese model applies to latent causation for actual events or as a preventative model for potential errors. This means that Choice *D* is incorrect.

**27. B:** The AHRQ is responsible for constructing and publishing current patient safety quality indicators (PSIs) that refer to adverse events during inpatient care. The majority of the current PSIs relate to avoidable maternal-child and perioperative complications. The remaining PSIs address a variety of conditions that may not have a specific hospital-related etiology, such as iatrogenic pneumothorax. The ER admission for an injury sustained before admission is not a PSI, which means that Choice *A* is incorrect. However, hip fractures resulting from falls by inpatients are a current PSI. Infiltration of IV solution into the surrounding tissue is a common occurrence that is not identified as a PSI, which means that Choice *C* is incorrect. In contrast, however, infections of central venous catheter IV sites that result in sepsis are tracked as a PSI. An infection contracted outside of the hospital is not tracked as a PSI, which means that Choice *D* is incorrect.

**28. B:** Reason believed that error assessment had to go beyond questioning the issues at the sharp end of the error to include the issues at the blunt end. Choice *B* is correct because the nurse committed the med error (the sharp end); however, the investigation needs to include the contributing factors that are at the blunt end of the error. Choices *A, C*, and *D* are incorrect because they each identify a latent cause that contributed to an error.

**29. D:** Identification of stakeholders is not an element of the Work Breakdown Structure (WBS), which is focused on the performance evaluation of deliverables. Therefore, Choice *D* is correct. The remaining choices—deliverables, tasks, and work packages—are all included in the work breakdown structure, making Choices *A, B*, and *C* incorrect.

**30. C:** HIPAA does not require encryption of PHI data, and there is no financial incentive for providing encryption. Hospitals are required to inform patients that PHI is not encrypted if patients request its transfer via email. Choices *A* and *B* are incorrect because agency data backup plans and mobile device usage plans are required for HIPAA compliance and would be included in a risk assessment test.

Organizations often fail to document the use of the safety measures associated with PHI. Hospitals often comply with all safety measures but fail the risk assessment because the documentation is incomplete. Therefore, Choice *D* is also incorrect.

**31. D:** The Systems Engineering Initiative for Patient Safety (SEIPS) addresses the relationships among work systems, work processes, and the outcomes associated with both. The initiative was commissioned by the AHRQ to broaden the scope of the patient safety models. The system uses many of the common assessment measures to evaluate the effects of ergonomic engineering on employee work performance, identify the effects of environmental conditions on patient safety, and assess the effectiveness of quality improvement efforts. The environmental factors associated with SEIPS include physical factors such as noise and lightening, socio-organizational factors such as management structure, and external factors such as societal and political position. This means that Choice *A* is incorrect. The people factor refers to patients and employees. Safety outcomes for both groups are addressed in the plan. That means that Choice *B* is incorrect. The model is based on human factors and ergonomics framework, which means that Choice *C* is incorrect.

**32. D:** CMS does not require that sentinel events be reported; however, CMS does require the healthcare organization to have a detailed plan for the entire root cause analysis procedure for any untoward event. The agency-generated incident report is used to document all details of the incident. This report is not added to the patient's record, but the information is discoverable in the event of any legal action. The FDA does not require but does encourage voluntary reporting in part to support the credibility of the patient-oriented drug information dashboard. This means that Choice *D* is correct.

**33. A:** Reciprocity bias occurs when a team member who has received a positive evaluation gives every other member of the team a positive evaluation that may or may not be valid. Choice *B* is an example of the halo bias wherein Jack thinks that since the project was successful, the whole team was successful as well. This means that Choice *B* is incorrect. Fred's evaluation is an example of inflation bias, which may affect the individual performance scores. This means that Choice *C* is incorrect. Ann's evaluation is an example of scapegoating bias, which generally occurs when the project has been unsuccessful. This means that Choice *D* is incorrect.

**34. B:** The Supreme Court ruling in National Federation of Independent Business v. Sebelius gave individual states the option of adopting the new eligibility rules. States are not required to adopt the rules, making Choice *A* incorrect. The new eligibility requirements applied to adults, not children, which means that Choice *C* is incorrect. Currently, thirty-five states have voluntarily expanded Medicaid coverage to adults who meet the revised standard, which means that Choice *D* is incorrect.

**35. C:** The modified SWOT framework provides the opportunity for the employee to self-evaluate strengths and areas for improvement. These comments also provide the manager with insights as to the need for additional resources to improve employee performance in general. This means that Choice *C* is correct. Choice *A* is incorrect because the employee agreed to the employee/employer contract that identifies the criteria for performance evaluation, so this means that the employee can challenge the results of the evaluation but cannot challenge the criteria for the evaluation. Choice *B* is incorrect because the performance appraisal is not an adversarial process. Choice *D* is incorrect because the framework is being used to evaluate the performance of one employee.

**36. A:** The Core Quality Measures Collaborative (CQMC) is a large group of interested parties convened by CMS to address the ever-expanding volume of work required for external reporting by providers of all

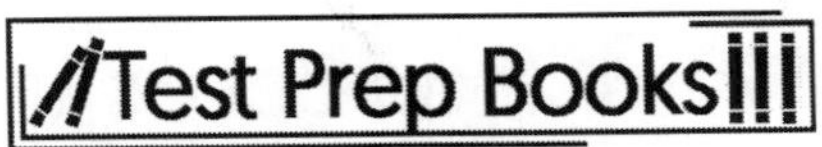

types. The group includes hospitals, insurers, ambulatory care, and long-term providers; private and group home physicians; and additional interested individuals. The collaborative focused on streamlining all regulatory reporting that addresses compliance with the core measures. The move to value-based care outcomes makes this work even more critical. Currently, the focus of the group is the evaluation of the ways that each of the core outcomes addresses disparities in the provision of care. The post-pandemic recommendations would more likely be issued by the CDC than CMS, which means that Choice *B* is incorrect. There are existing core measures that address antibiotic management; however, the current focus of the workgroup is addressing disparities in care, which means that Choice *C* is incorrect. Establishing emergency care protocols is beyond the scope of the workgroup, making Choice *D* is incorrect.

**37. A:** The basic requirement of systems thinking is the understanding that connections among all departments need to be identified and evaluated as the basis for successful risk reduction for the entire system. Fixing a faulty process in the laboratory will fail unless the impact of the new process on the nursing units, transportation services, and technology services is included in the plan. That means that Choice *A* is correct. Systems thinking is effective because it is a non-linear process that responds to the complexities of the system. Choice *B* is incorrect because systems thinking would recognize that a unit-specific assessment would be required. As noted, systems thinking looks at all the parts of the whole system, and that means that Choice *C* is incorrect. The literature suggests that systems thinking is essential for smaller systems to evaluate risk-potential as the systems expands, so that means that Choice *D* is incorrect.

**38. B:** Using only the patient portal to announce the program is a process error because patients covered by Medicare are generally over the age of 65 and may or may not be computer savvy or have internet access. The team made an assumption that potentially limited the effectiveness of the plan, which means that Choice *B* is correct. Choice *A* is a project outcome rather than a process error which means that Choice *A* is incorrect. Choices *C* and *D* are incorrect because they are both environmental failure effects rather than process effects.

**39. A:** The focus of Clinical Effectiveness Research (CER) is to support rigorous research protocols that compare and contrast proposed treatment options and disseminate those results to care providers. CER designs can include both quantitative and qualitative designs, so Choice *B* is incorrect. The original intent of CER is focused on specific diseases, rather than population-based issues such as water and food supply resources for underserved nations. This means that Choice *C* is incorrect. CER provides funding for small and large studies. The important design element is the identification and comparison of possible interventions rather than the size of the research group, which means that Choice *D* is incorrect.

**40. C:** The HEDIS database compiles disease-specific information for each of the listed domains except the cumulative costs of care. The domains of the HEDIS database documentation include care effectiveness, care accessibility and access, the patient-care experience, risk-adjusted utilization, health plans' descriptive information, and details of electronic data system use. That means that Choices *A, B*, and *D* are incorrect.

**41. C:** The original Magnet plan was based on fourteen Forces of Magnetism (FOM) that were incorporated into four elements of nursing excellence. In 2008, the American Nurses Credentialing Center (ANCC) added the reporting of performance outcomes related to professional practice and research as the fifth critical criterion for certification. Choices *A, B,* and *D* were each included in the original elements of nursing excellence, which means that they are incorrect.

**42. A:** The quote "significant few - trivial many" as applied to project planning refers to the fact that eighty percent of the problems can be traced to just twenty percent of the identified causes, which is often depicted in a PARETO analysis. This means that Choice *A* is correct. An environmental cause of FMEA analysis would be an avoidable natural event such as a hurricane that affected the project outcome, which means that Choice *B* is incorrect. Choice *C* is incorrect because it is comparing two variables rather than analyzing cause and effect. The development of the fishbone diagram is often recommended as the preliminary step of PARETO analysis, which means that Choice *D* is incorrect.

**43. B:** The Medicare Health Outcomes Survey (HOS) uses the HEDIS database information to evaluate patient care as the basis for Star Ratings that are awarded for excellent provider care. Each year, CMS identifies three HEDIS effectiveness-of-care measures for the current report. Consumers can use the report to add context to the star ratings, and CMS can use the data to evaluate customer satisfaction. The current reporting measures include assessment of physical activity, bladder control management, and fall-risk reduction. The survey is completed by a random sample of Medicare recipients, which may or may not be over 65, because Medicare coverage is extended to patients under the age of 65 with various disabilities. This means that Choice *A* is incorrect. The survey is completed by patients rather than providers or hospitals, which means that Choices *C* and *D* are incorrect.

**44. C:** Thought mapping is viewed as an essential first step. The process builds on the identification of the goals and scope of the improvement process to create a visual representation of the entire project. The map is not static; it is a workable guide that evolves as the DMAIC questions are answered. This means that Choice *C* is the correct answer. Choice *A* is incorrect because, by definition, the thought mapping process is a team effort. The team leader and team members define the process that is the best fit for the project purpose and goals; therefore, Choice *B* is incorrect. One of the essential outcomes of the mind mapping process is the prioritized list of questions to be addressed in the DMAIC protocol, which means that Choice *D* is incorrect.

**45. B:** The NCQA provides certification for individual providers, provider groups, and healthcare plans. The certification is based on clinical performance outcomes and consumer satisfaction, which is unique to this organization. Health-plan performance reporting is widely used by employers and consumers to evaluate and choose health plans. The Joint Commission on Accreditation of Healthcare Organizations (JCAHO) is a private, non-profit organization that accredits hospitals, outpatient surgical centers, and laboratories. Patient outcomes, rather than consumer satisfaction, are the basis for JCAHO accreditation, which means that Choice *A* is incorrect. The Utilization Review Accreditation Commission (URAC) accredits those healthcare agencies that demonstrate commitment to rigorous review and reporting of all quality-of-care data. The review standards do not address consumer experiences, which means that Choice *C* is incorrect. The American Association for Ambulatory Health Care (AAAHC) accredits ambulatory care centers that provide evidence of ongoing staff development programs, self-evaluation, and peer review activities. These criteria are not associated with consumer feedback, which means that Choice *D* is incorrect.

**46. C:** Human factors engineering analyzes how individuals use technology to identify potential areas of risk. Individuals develop a work-around when the designated process doesn't work. For instance, at one point, the barcoding system did not consistently scan IV bags. This system failure led to the work-around where nurses started the infusion and then documented the solution in the EHR, bypassing the proper

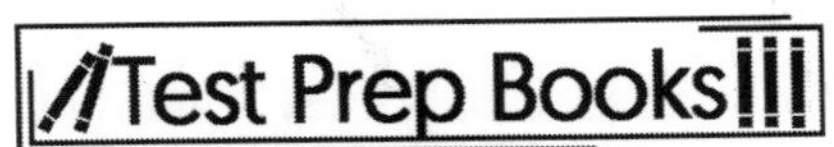

identification of the solution. This particular work-around resulted in patient deaths. The manufacturers have since increased the sensitivity of the scanners and high-risk IV solutions containing anesthetic agents, heparin, and potassium have enhanced safety requirements. Human factors engineers understand that the human factor will remain, but these security refinements are aimed at decreasing the incidence of untoward events. This means that Choice *C* is the correct answer. Choice *A* is incorrect because, by definition, the work-around bypasses safeguards and increases the risk for harm. Choice *B* is incorrect because the time saved in a work-around is proportionate to the increased risk of the procedure which is not a desirable outcome. Choice *D* is incorrect because the work-around is a behavior rather than the analysis of a process.

**47. C:** Validation confirms that the completed outcomes of the process improvement protocol will solve the original problem. This means that Choice *C* is correct. Choice *A* is the definition of *verification*, which indicates that the identified solution is appropriate to the selected outcomes. Therefore, Choice *A* is incorrect. Validation is not specifically related to "gaps" in the knowns or the selection of Six Sigma tools, which means that Choices *B* and *D* are incorrect.

**48. A:** Although both prescriptive and predictive analytical methods provide a view of future outcomes based on past performance, prescriptive analytical methods use advanced analytical algorithms to provide an action plan to match the predictions. In other words, predictive analytics would provide the team with a picture of the care unit going forward, while prescriptive analytics would describe the future view and a specific plan for how to achieve the successes identified in that view. This means that Choice *B* is incorrect. Descriptive analytics looks at historical and current data to identify relationships and trends data; however, these simple calculations are not predictive of future outcomes, so Choice *C* is incorrect. Diagnostic analytics are used for root cause analysis rather than predicting the future, which means that Choice *D* is incorrect.

**49. D:** The International Standards Organization (ISO) sets standards; however, an independent review of the agency's compliance with each standard is required for certification. This means that the independent auditor, not the ISO, confers the certification. ISO standard compliance is voluntary and not associated with CMS standards, which means that Choice *A* is incorrect. There is no hierarchy of standards, and quality standards from accrediting agencies frequently overlap, which means that Choice *B* is incorrect. Certification for the ISO standards must be renewed every 3 years, so Choice *D* is incorrect.

**50. D:** All of the choices are examples of safeguards for the human factor-technology interface; however, the processes are associated with increased error risk. In contrast, physically removing the KCl vials decreases the human factor to a greater degree than the remaining choices. A nurse cannot add too much KCl to the bag if the nurse doesn't have a vial of KCl. The manufacturers responded by providing pre-mixed IV solutions with standardized concentrations of KCl. Choice *A* is incorrect because more than one dose can be given. Choice *B* is incorrect because drug diversion and administration errors are still possible. Choice *C* is incorrect because even though CPOE has substantially decreased the error risk, risks associated with time delays and incorrect entries remain.

**51. A:** Choice *A* is the correct answer because the work package contains all the process and content details of the deliverables. The remaining choices influence the identification of the deliverables; however, the project outcomes, the KPIs, and the scope of the process are not included in an individual work package. This means that Choices *B, C,* and *D* are incorrect.

**52. A:** The National Institute of Standards and Technologies, a division of the United States Department of Commerce, is responsible for the Baldrige Award. This award for organizational excellence sets standards and evaluates compliance in all business environments including healthcare. The intent of the award is to establish and maintain the competitive edge of American businesses. The standards are industry-specific, and only the most successful organizations achieve the award. Healthcare leaders are increasingly challenged to protect the market share of the organization because maintaining the reputation of the hospital is essential to the financial health of an institution. Even in smaller healthcare markets, some of the identified disruptive technologies such as telehealth, minute clinics, and concierge care models can affect the bottom line of a hospital. This means that Choices *B, C*, and *D* need to be addressed to achieve the ultimate goal of protecting the hospital's reputation.

**53. D:** In 2017, the Food and Drug Administration (FDA) implemented the Digital Health Innovation Action Plan that provides a detailed product review of AI "devices" for healthcare applications. CMS reimbursement decisions are based on these certification reviews by the FDA. Currently, there are several specific CMS reimbursement schedules for AI implementation, including the Medicare Physician Fee Schedule (MPFS) and the Outpatient Prospective Payment System (OPPS) for the IDx-DR system. CMS also reimburses the Viz LVO systems costs for stroke detection and cardiac ultrasound in the New Technology Add-on Payments (NTAP) in the Inpatient Prospective Payment System (IPPS). This means that Choice *A* is incorrect. There is a select number of radiology studies that are currently reimbursed by CMS such as the previously mentioned Viz LVO system for stroke detection; however, AI is not used for radiology studies. This means that Choice *B* is incorrect. The financial logistics of AI implementation currently do not include single-use patient charges for AI interventions. In other words, if an AI system is used to diagnose a patient's stroke, the patient is not currently charged for the costs of the AI system. So, Choice *C* is incorrect.

**54. D:** High-reliability healthcare systems maintain a proactive anticipatory mindset for risk reduction, which means that Choice *D* is the correct answer. Choices *A, B,* and *C* are incorrect because they each identify one characteristic of the high-reliability healthcare systems.

**55. D**: Six Sigma methodology suggests that in order to identify the actual cost versus benefit of a proposed solution, frequent analysis is required at several points in the process rather than at a single point in the process. This means that Choice *D* is correct because it includes the remaining choices. Choices *A, B*, and *C* are incorrect because limiting the cost-benefit analysis to any single point in the process would not account for gaps in the process at other points.

**56. C:** The Commission on Accreditation of Rehabilitation Facilities (CARF) maintains a comprehensive website that includes a searchable database of agencies with current accreditation. Consumers can use search filters to identify accredited services in the United States and Canada. It is a private non-profit organization, so Choice *A* is incorrect. Third-party payers use the accreditation information to estimate the risks and benefits of covering care in an accredited facility; however, accreditation is not a requirement for coverage of care. Therefore, Choice *B* is incorrect. Agencies that provide care across the life span are eligible for CARF accreditation. For instance, accreditation standards are set for organizations that provide aging services, child and youth services, and opioid rehabilitation services. This means that Choice *D* is incorrect.

**57. A:** Choice *A* is the correct answer because innovators are the first to possess the new device or have access to the latest technology. Choice *B* is incorrect because early adopters are leaders who will consider the price of the watch, but they don't base their purchase decisions on public opinion.

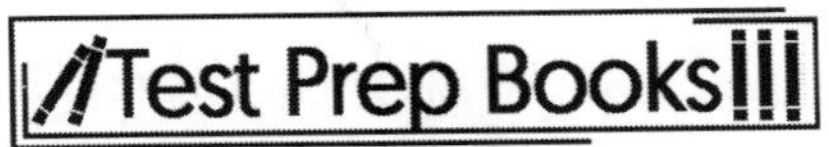

Innovators do not consider the cost of the watch; they buy the watch because it the first of its kind, so Choice *C* is incorrect. The early majority members, not the early adopters, wait to read about all the watch's details. This means that Choice *D* is incorrect.

**58. B:** The Fast Healthcare Interoperability Resource (FHIR) standards are used to promote the development of applications that facilitate the interchange of data across systems. Industry experts predict that these "apps" will successfully address the long-standing problem associated with the development and use of EHR systems. These applications are expected to address multiple uses of EHR data, including chronic disease management and provider dashboard improvements; however, the patients will most likely notice that there is no longer a need for multiple patient portals as a result of the data integration. This means that Choices *A, C,* and *D* are incorrect.

**59. B:** All accreditations ultimately affect the bottom line; however, JCAHO accreditation is required for CMS reimbursement, which means that it should be the priority for team leaders. Magnet status requires three years of documentation before accreditation, so while planning is required, the accreditation will not address immediate concerns. Therefore, Choice *A* is incorrect. The ISO accreditation and the Baldrige Award would also be included in long-range planning because the accreditations are dependent on a history of organizational excellence. That means that Choices *C* and *D* are incorrect.

**60. A:** The surgeon/provider is legally responsible for the identification of the appropriate operative site—arm, leg, fingers, toes, etc. However, the actual signing can be delegated to a licensed person with post-graduate education such as the NP or PA who works with the surgeon and is therefore acquainted with the patient.

**61. B:** Choice *B* is correct because a value stream map is used in the *measure* step of the DMAIC method to assess the current status of the project. The *define* step uses a process map to identify the success of the process improvement, meaning that Choice *A* is incorrect. Choice *C* is incorrect because the *analyze* step uses cause and effect instruments such as the fishbone diagram to track changes in the project. The *improve* step uses process maps to compare the existing model with the proposed model, which means that Choice *D* is incorrect.

**62. D:** The CQMC identified the Quality Core Measures to be used to effectively document quality patient care. The work was directed at removing redundant measures or measures that were not reliability collecting quality data as well as new measures that specifically addressed value-based care reporting. The core measures were developed for private and government-funded payers, which means that Choice *A* is incorrect. The measures were specifically chosen to facilitate documentation of value-based care, so Choice *B* is incorrect. Measures that address care costs are included in the core measures, so Choice *C* is incorrect.

**63. A:** The JCAHO Survey Analysis for Evaluating Risk Matrix (SAFER Matrix) is a visual representation of the degree of risk and the scope of the error associated with each Requirement for Improvement (RFI). The degree of risk to patients, hospital staff, and visitors is scored as low, medium, or high. The scope of each RFI is scored as limited occurrences, exhibiting a pattern, or being widespread.

Agencies must submit the Evidence of Standards Compliance (ESC) documentation to identify efforts to improve processes and prevent future occurrences within sixty days of receipt of the JCAHO analysis. This means that Choice *B* is incorrect. The matrix addresses the scope of the area of non-compliance rather than the number of times the error is made. For instance, if an error only occurs in Department X, even if Department X makes the error one hundred times, the risk is limited to that department. If the same error occurs in a pattern or is widespread across the agency, the risk of harm increases. This means that Choice *C* is incorrect. The most critical RFIs include high-risk compliance errors that are widespread across the agency. The JCAHO visitors can choose to focus on these items in subsequent visits; however, the review of low-risk RFIs is limited to the submission of the ESC plan for improvement and prevention. This means that Choice *D* is incorrect.

**64. B:** Six Sigma is a powerful management system that is most effective in companies that employ standard measures for process assessment and improvement. Systems that use more creative assessment procedures are encouraged to explore systems that support their needs, such as the waterfall methodology that separates the steps of the creative process into separate categories for process assessment. This means that Choice *B* is correct because Six Sigma is designed for the standard steps of the manufacturing process. The Children's Art School and the AI Software company would have different needs for process assessment that could be better addressed by an alternative methodology, which means that Choices *A* and *D* are incorrect. Choice *C* is incorrect because healthcare organizations require patient care assessments that are different than the process assessments at the Widget company.

**65. C:** Handwashing is the essential first step in preventing hospital-acquired infections. Choices *A, B*, and *D* are important parts of the overall patient safety, but the 2022 guidelines specially address handwashing. This means that Choice *C* is correct.

**66. D:** Workers' Compensation insurance does provide financial support for injured employees; however, the Occupational Safety and Health Administration (OSHA) is not associated with any aspect of the compensation plan. The OSHA standards address the safety issues related to the care of potentially violent patients, which means that Choice *A* is incorrect. Healthcare workers sustain injuries at three times the national average for other industries. Most of these injuries are musculoskeletal injuries that can be avoided with the use of mechanical aids to transfer patients. The financial investment in mechanical lift systems is returned by decreased employee injuries, increased patient safety related to falls and skin injuries, and increased patient satisfaction. This means that Choice *B* is incorrect. There are OSHA standards aimed at decreasing the risk of contamination such as the use of personal protective equipment (PPE), which means that Choice *C* is incorrect.

**67. A:** Mistake proofing is a six-step method of addressing possible process errors before the implementation of the plan. Facilitation is focused on making the process step easier to decrease errors. For instance, in a task with multiple wires to be connected, color coding the individual wires according to their function will speed production. Facilitation is used most often because simple adjustments to any process increase team efficiency, meaning that Choice *A* is correct. Choice *B* is incorrect because elimination refers to the removal of a potential error rather than the modification of the system. Replacement refers to switching elements of the design process to avoid potential errors, so Choice *C* is incorrect. Mitigation addresses decreasing the impact of the process error once it occurs, which means that Choice *D* is incorrect as well.

**68. B:** The Consumers Assessment of Healthcare Providers and Systems (CAHPS) survey reveals important consumer satisfaction information for every aspect of the patient's healthcare experience. The resulting survey data can be used by providers to identify areas for improvement, measure the success of quality improvement efforts, and provide competitive benchmarks. The AHRQ developed the

CAHPS and provides researchers with detailed information for the use of this trademarked survey; however, there is no fee for use of the data. This means that Choice *A* is incorrect. Use of the CAHPS survey is voluntary, but providers can use the data to assess patient satisfaction as noted above. This means that Choice *C* is incorrect. The CAHPS survey measures all aspects of the patient's experience with hospitals, primary and specialty care providers, and office staff. This means that Choice *D* is incorrect.

**69. C:** Choice *C* is correct because the qualitative approach of the GPS plan would allow the manager to identify company support strategies that could improve individual performance and decrease employee turnover rates. Choice *A* is incorrect because the qualitative approach will result in better management/employee relations and will also free the manager from defending the numerical system, which is a one-size-fits-all approach to human behavior. Choice *B* is incorrect because the focus of the PIP is not punitive. It is a positive model designed to strengthen employee performance by identifying a plan for growth potential. Choice *D* is incorrect because the GPS plan could increase the number of rewards due to a more accurate performance assessment.

**70. B:** The processing time for insurance claims is designated as a key financial performance indicator. Although the bed turnover rate ultimately affects the financial status of the hospital, the rate is identified as a patient-care performance indicator, which means that Choice *A* is incorrect. The average radiology department wait time is also considered a patient-care performance indicator because it addresses patient satisfaction and staff performance. This means that Choice *C* is incorrect. The utilization documentation for medical equipment would be found in the nursing notes of the EHR, which means that the performance indicator is a patient-care metric rather than a financial metric. Therefore, Choice *D* is incorrect.

**71. A:** Internal and competitive benchmarking is a cost-effective way to identify hospital procedures and processes that are not contributing value to the organization. Experts caution team leaders that benchmarking results alone is not a roadmap for fixing the process. This means that Choice *B* is incorrect. There is a tendency for success to foster complacency. This means that if an institution is meeting every internal and competitor benchmark, the impetus for innovation can be negatively affected. This means that Choice *C* is incorrect. If the wrong types of benchmarking data are used to evaluate a process, time and effort will be wasted on process improvements. This means that Choice *D* is incorrect.

**72. C:** The cost-benefit analysis may generate decisions that will benefit the company but may not always coincide with the humanistic response to the issue. For instance, it would benefit the company to eliminate the $100 employee reward for a gym membership. The company would save money, but employees have less incentive to pursue healthy choices at the gym. Choice *C* is the correct answer because although the humanistic approach would be to continue offering the reward, the business decision could be to discontinue the benefit. This conflict could be difficult for some members of the team. The completed cost-benefit analysis is based on objective data, and it also can identify hidden elements of the financial plan that have not been previously discussed. This means that Choices *A, B,* and *D* are incorrect.

**73. C:** When the Lean Six Sigma methodology is applied in a healthcare system, the end product is *control* of inherent risks, which means that Choice *C* is correct. The remaining choices are potential by-products of the Lean Six Sigma process; however, managing patient risk is the primary goal. Choices *A* and *B* could be improved by controlling the wastes that are identified in the DMAIC process, and Choice *D* could result from improved patient outcomes that translate to improved patient satisfaction.

**74. D:** The National Special Pathogen System of Care (NSPS) model includes the use of a Central Body to promote standardization and coordinate care for this four-tiered approach to patient and community care in the event of the emergence of another pathogen. Tier A facilities can provide high-level isolation care for pediatric and adult patients while coordinating care among regional Tier B, C, and D facilities. Tier B facilities can provide comprehensive care for large numbers of patients. Tier C facilities can provide rapid testing and advanced care for special pathogens such as Ebola for large numbers of patients.

Tier D facilities include most acute-care facilities in the United States that provide basic pathogen isolation and care procedures. There will be an estimated ten to twenty Tier A facilities in the United States once the plan is fully implemented. The NSPS model is federally funded and was developed by the National Emerging Special Pathogens Training and Education Center (NETEC), which is a division of the HHS Office of the Assistant Secretary for Preparedness and Response. This means that Choice *A* is incorrect. Participation is not voluntary, which means that Choice *B* is incorrect. Choice *C* is incorrect because the Central Body will assign facilities to different tier levels according to the ability to provide specialized care for infectious diseases.

**75. D:** Choice *D* is correct because the early adopters are often leaders whose implementation of new processes and products influences the implementation behavior of others. Choice *A* is incorrect because the laggards won't influence anyone since they are very slow to adopt the innovation. Choice *B* is incorrect because the late majority remains skeptical about the innovation even after others have adopted the innovation. Choice *C* is incorrect because although the early majority will implement the new process before the average person, the members of this group are less likely to be influential leaders.

**76. A:** According to the Lean Six Sigma methodology, the "eighth" waste is the lost human potential that results from the combined effects of the identified wastes. When the wastes are controlled, individual performance improves. Choice *B* is incorrect because excess motion in healthcare systems refers to the misuse of ergonomics in activities such as moving patients from one bed to another bed. This is an area of personal vulnerability for all patient care employees. Choice *C* is incorrect because over processing refers to minimizing procedures such as "paperwork". This waste is often the result of EHR programming that requires redundant data entry. Choice *D,* wait times, is part of the problem but since it is the seventh waste, this choice is incorrect.

**77. A:** Large portions of EHR data entry exist in a narrative form that requires translation before the data can be processed and reported. Although AI systems such as machine learning and natural language processing systems are being developed, narrative data translation continues to be a major barrier to cross-system communication. The cost of AI machine learning software resources that are approved by the FDA by individual providers is reimbursed by CMS, which means that Choice *B* is incorrect. The human input time is decreased with the use of AI innovations, so Choice *C* is incorrect. Machine learning produces data-entry procedures that save time and improve the quality and accuracy of the data entries, which supports improved patient-care outcomes. This means that Choice *D* is incorrect.

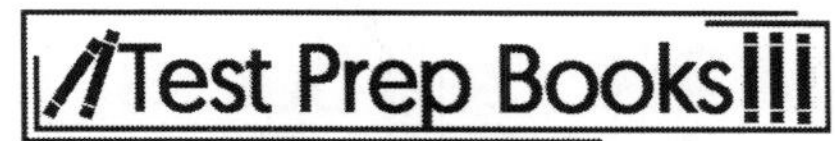

**78. C:** The goals of the NSPS model include zero preventable deaths, mobilization of the care network within two hours of notification of the risk, and one hundred percent patient access to care. The remaining choices do not list the goals of the NSPS models.

**79. A:** The GR&R measures the variation in performance for repeated measurements under identical conditions. In the example, hypothetically, one measure of the final product might be the voltage. Any variation in the voltage over several trials with the same person operating the same testing equipment will be identified in the GR&R test. Choice *A* is correct because the GR&R results will be compared to acceptable variation limits for the voltage of the pacemaker to determine the success of the proposed innovation. Choice *B* is incorrect because stakeholder satisfaction or the voice of the customer is captured in opinion surveys, interviews, or focus groups, and the results are used in the earlier planning stages of the Six Sigma plan. Choice *C* is incorrect because root cause analysis is determined with measures such fishbone diagrams, PARETO charts, and the FMEA measure, and it is focused on the causes for variation rather than determining the amount of process variation as in the GR&R test. The determination of the sample size is required for the pilot study that tests the success of the QI intervention, meaning that Choice *D* is incorrect.

**80. D:** The 5S process organizes the workplace to improve employee morale and performance. Each of the 5S steps is specific to one area of the workplace. An example of standardization is supplying every patient care area with the identical stock, which means that everyone knows what is and is not available on the unit. Ideally, the specific location would also be the same in all nursing units. This means that Choice *D* is the correct answer. Choice *A is* incorrect because environmental cleanliness is the focus of the third S: ***scrub***. Color coding patient care items is an example of straightening which decreases clutter and improves employee access to necessary items. That means that Choice *B* is incorrect. A clutter-free is an example of the *sort* step, which is the first step to an organized workplace, so Choice *C* is incorrect.

**81. A:** The details of all negative reviews are published, which means that insurers are aware of the error rates of an institution, and the increased risk can result in increased fees. The reports detail all non-compliance issues, which means that Choices *B* and *C* are incorrect. The evaluation of individual performance related to the review may be punitive in some instances, such as an error due to willful neglect of a standard for patient care. This means that Choice *D* is incorrect.

**82. C:** The IHI has defined the Triple Aim of healthcare delivery as a model for providing and reporting value-based care. The three areas of this initiative include population health, patient experience, and per capita care costs, and the IHI has identified specific metrics to document care for each of these areas. The Composite Health Risk Appraisal (HRA) score is a self-reported measure of the individual's health status related to nutrition, exercise, mental health, and biometric measures such as blood pressure and cholesterol levels. The results of the survey provide an individualized risk assessment that generates areas of improvement for the patient. The IHI recommends the use of this metric to address population health. The emergency department utilization is used to address the per capita costs, which means that Choice *A* is incorrect. The IOM Quality Chasm Assessment is used to assess the effectiveness and safety of health care delivery and to make recommendations for improvement. The IHI identifies this measure as an appropriate metric for assessing the patient experience aim. This means that Choice *B* is incorrect. The CAHPS global measure also addresses the patient experience, so Choice *D* is incorrect.

**83. B:** Six Sigma implementation commonly affects the product price. The product must be free of defects 99.9996 percent of the time, and the process improvements that are required to reach this goal commonly increase the price of production and the final cost of the product, so Choice *B* is correct. As a result of the cost of product improvements, company revenues decrease (at least initially); therefore, Choice *A* is incorrect. The basic principle of Six Sigma is that QI (quality improvement) is a continuous process that is required to maintain the gains from a single project. This means that Choice *C* is incorrect. If the Six Sigma methodology is introduced with the appropriate support from management and adequate educational preparation for all employees, then employee satisfaction typically increases because the model empowers employees to reach their leadership potential. Therefore, Choice *D* is incorrect.

**84. B:** The research indicates that failure to consider the sustainability of any quality improvement project will often result in the ultimate failure of the process. Team leaders are encouraged to communicate the ongoing success of the project and to invite participation in the continuous improvement model. Choice *A* is incorrect because the performance evaluation measure is part of the original implementation plan rather than the sustainability plan. Publishing the details of the successful innovation is important; however, the continued success of the innovation is the product of the sustainability plan, which means that Choice *C* is incorrect. The implementation plan is incomplete without the sustainability plan, which means that Choice *D* is incorrect.

**85. A:** Customer value-added activities are any costs of the product that are important and acceptable to the customer. In general, changes that have a positive effect on the customer's experience are considered value-added activities. Choice *A* is correct because decreased product delivery time is a direct benefit to the customer. Choice *B* is incorrect because redesigning the workstations directly benefits the company by improving production, which means that this redesign is a business value-added activity. Digitization of the inventory control is also a business value-added activity that directly benefits the company, which means that Choice *C* is incorrect. An evaluation of employee skills is also a business value-added activity because the results of the testing can evolve into better management decisions and less "waste" of employee talent as defined by Six Sigma. This means that Choice *D* is incorrect because it is a business value-added activity that won't directly affect the customers' experience.

**86. A:** A "never event' is defined as a serious reportable event (SRE) that causes harm and is most often preventable. Lists of these events have been compiled by the Joint Commission, the National Quality Forum, and other industry "watchdog" organizations such as LeapFrog. Reporting these events is mandatory in many states, while voluntary reporting to the Joint Commission is encouraged. Choice *A* is correct because serious harm is possible, and the event is preventable. Choice *B* can have significant consequences; however, it can occur even with proper care, which means that Choice *B* is incorrect. Choice *C* is a serious error; however, it occurred before admission to the hospital, which means it is not a never event. An IV site phlebitis generally resolves without harm and can occur even with proper care of the IV site, so Choice *D* is incorrect.

**87. D:** Porter's model addresses the market forces that affect a provider. The forces identified in this model include the threat of new entrants, buyer power, supplier power, the threat of substitutes, and the threat of rivalry. This business-oriented framework is also useful for healthcare providers. The new eye-care group will need to address the barriers facing new marketplace entrants. The start-up technology costs for eye-care specialists are substantial, and as new providers, the group will need to continually update the technology to remain competitive, which means that Choice *A* is correct. The scope of the healthcare environment is no longer local because novel care practices such as medical tourism have increased the competition, so Choice *B* is correct. The concept of "brand loyalty" differentiates healthcare models from business models. Overcoming the existing provider-patient

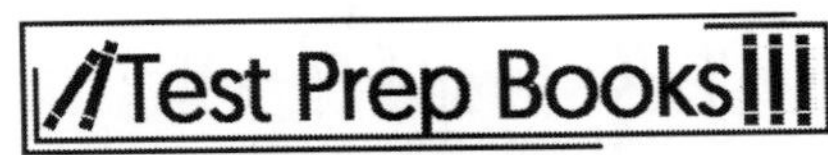

relationship is more difficult for new groups than conquering the "Coke or Pepsi" challenge. This means that Choice *C* is also correct.

**88. D:** A balanced scorecard is used to map company strategy in four areas: customer service, finances, internal business, and learning and growth. The balanced scorecard is used in companies of all sizes, but it is viewed as an essential exercise for senior management in large companies, which means that Choice *D* is the correct answer. The remaining choices correctly identify attributes of the balanced scorecard, so Choices *A, B*, and *C* are incorrect.

**89. C:** The Quality Compass provides trended reports for the comparison of institutional data with HEDIS database information and CAHPS consumer data. This analysis uses internal benchmarking data, not competitive data, so Choice *A* is incorrect. The measure provides a detailed analysis rather than a checklist, which means that Choice *B* is incorrect. The Quality Compass data is used by hospital team leaders to assess institutional performance, and the results are not reported to anyone outside of the institution. This means that Choice *D* is incorrect.

**90. B:** Choice *B* is correct because a cohesive team is committed to the project, demonstrates respect for individual opinions and talents, and communicates effectively as a team. Choice *A* is incorrect because cohesion develops when the team considers input from all individual team members; it does not require them all to agree completely. Choice *C* is incorrect because the team members create team cohesiveness. The leader presents the objectives for the project, but the group of individual team members evolves into a cohesive team because of mutual trust and focus on the success of the project. A group of motivated individuals does not immediately constitute a cohesive team. There will be conflicts and much discussion among team members on the path to becoming a cohesive team. This means that Choice *D* is incorrect because the cohesive team has moved beyond the forming stage by resolving the conflicts of the storming stage.

**91. C:** FMEA severity ratings are used to determine the characteristics of the event concerning the duration of the effect of the error, the need for additional care, and the likelihood that the error will prompt revision of the process associated with the error. Choice *C* is the correct answer because level 3 or moderately severe outcomes can prompt revision of the process to prevent future errors, and level 2 or minor occurrences do not promptly process revisions. Choice *A* is incorrect because level 3 occurrences are not reportable since they do not involve permanent harm. Choice *B* is incorrect because level 2 occurrences are minor and temporary and therefore do not require additional care. Choice *D* is incorrect because level 2 occurrences are minor and unpredictable.

**92. A:** America's Health Insurance Plans (AHIP) publishes core measures of excellence across nine specialties. The core measures are reviewed annually to remove measures that do not contribute to meaningful measures of value-based care and to add measures that address emerging measurement needs, such as equitable access to care and telehealth strategies. The measures are intended for use by ambulatory care providers such as individual practitioners, physician groups, and patient-centered medical homes to demonstrate the quality of care. The core measures relate to patient-care outcomes rather than self-report surveys, which means that Choice *B* is incorrect. The use of the core measures for care outcomes evaluation is voluntary and up to the discretion of the provider. This means that Choice *C* is incorrect. The core measures are designed to demonstrate patient-care outcomes in ambulatory settings rather than acute-care settings, which means that Choice *D* is incorrect.

**93. C:** The Accrediting Council for Continuing Medical Education (ACME) sets standards for programs that provide continuing medical education. Physicians are required to complete a specific number of continuing education units (CEUs) for license renewal, and the state medical boards can request the accreditation status of those hours. Program providers submit the detailed course outline to ACME, and approved plans can offer CEUs for completion of the course. Acceptable course content can be related to population health, skills performance, or research initiatives; however, CMS accreditation is not a function of ACME. This means that Choice *A* is incorrect. ACME sets standards for educational programs but does not track individual participation in those offerings, so Choice *B* is incorrect. Medical students would benefit educationally from the programs; however, as prelicensure students, CEUs are not required, which means that Choice *D* is incorrect.

**94. C:** In the implementation step, the person has already decided to accept the new idea but now must decide if it truly is helpful. This means that Choice *C* is correct. During the persuasion step, the person considers the idea and looks for additional information, so Choice *A* is incorrect. In the decision step, the person assesses the pros and cons of the new idea and decides to use it, so Choice *B* is incorrect. In the confirmation step, the person decides whether to continue using the new idea, so Choice *D* is incorrect.

**95. B:** Enterprise Management Software (EMS) programs are used to coordinate the business functions of an institution rather than the patient-care functions. Human Resources management is consistent with this business model. RCM software is designed to create maintenance and backup plans for critical systems such as heating and cooling, internet and phone services, and power. This means that Choice *A* is incorrect. Healthcare Customer Relations software measures patient satisfaction based on input from many sources that might include social media entries or EHR data. This information is not related to the use of enterprise-level data, so Choice *C* is incorrect. Individual patient data management is not addressed by EMS, which means that Choice *D* is incorrect.

**96. B:** AHRQ in-hospital quality indicators are associated with "never events" that should never occur. Institutions that successfully prevent pressure ulcers, central line infections, and sepsis have met the quality indicator. Although improved patient satisfaction may result from the hospital's success in preventing the never events, the focus of the quality indicators is prevention. This means that Choice *A* is incorrect. Accurate CMS reimbursement also can result from meeting the quality indicators; however, it is not the primary focus, which means that Choice *C* is incorrect. Failure to meet the quality indicators may result in the evaluation of staff performance, but the in-hospital quality indicators are patient-oriented. This means that Choice *D* is incorrect.

**97. D:** Defining the scope of the project is the essential first step of process improvement efforts. The critical elements of scope include the suppliers, input, process, output, and customers. The distribution plan is not part of the scope of the project, so Choice *D* is correct. The suppliers for all required project resources are identified in the process map for the project scope, which means that Choice *A* is incorrect. Choice *B* is incorrect because the process is defined as all the steps that are required to move the project from the raw materials to the finished project. Choice *C* is also incorrect because the widget is the output of the project, and it is an essential element of the project scope.

**98. A:** Bundled care payments are based on an episode of care. Providers and hospitals are reimbursed a set fee for care related to a clinical encounter, and this financial responsibility ends ninety days after the patient is discharged or after the procedure. This model transfers financial risk to the provider. If the actual cost of care is less than the set fee, the providers receive a financial reward. The cost of care for medical patients is generally greater than the costs for surgical patients because of the common readmission rate for chronic diseases. This means that Choice *B* is incorrect. As noted, providers are required to repay only portions of the sustained losses, which means that Choice *C* is incorrect. Surgical patient charges for SNF care increase the costs, and one of the ways providers manage costs is to transfer the patient to home care rather than SNF. This means that Choice *D* is incorrect.

**99. C:** Choice *C* is correct because additional stress on the individual team members is a characteristic of *muri*, which could be caused by any of the seven common faults. For instance, if there weren't proper educational resources for the employee or proper tools for the job, errors would be more likely. The errors would translate to additional stress on the individual and added work hours to replace defective products. Choice *A* is incorrect because variations in production are defined as *mura* in the Toyota model. As mentioned, *mura* is commonly due to one of the common faults. An example would be if the inventory weren't properly managed, then the weekly production totals would vary from week to week depending on the availability of the resource materials. This same inventory fault could also increase the production cost per unit, which is another example of *mura*. This means that Choice *B* is incorrect. Choice *D* is incorrect because negative customer feedback is an example of one of the seven wastes that define *muda*.

**100. A:** The SEMOS measure evaluates the initial results of the specific sentinel event action plan and is then used to provide periodic checks on the plan's effectiveness. Reporting of the event requires would include all of the clinical elements of the sentinel event and a detailed analysis of the effects of the error including root cause determination, which means that Choice *A* is correct. Choice *B* is incorrect because the report does not include an analysis of the results of the action plan. Choice *C* is incorrect because the plan does not address near-misses. Choice *D* is incorrect because the SEMOS addresses the action plan that is based on the root cause analysis.

**101. C:** The fishbone chart would provide the nurses with a root cause analysis framework to investigate the reasons for the increase. The remaining choices would provide other forms of information that could assess any changes in the central IV site care protocol. The run chart would display evidence of sustained improvement of changes in the protocol over time. The histogram would provide values of central tendency. The Pareto chart could identify areas of the process with great potential for improvement. This means that Choice *A, B,* and *D* are incorrect.

**102. C:** Pareto charts pinpoint areas that require review, which are identified as the vital few, as well as services that are meeting the patients' needs, which are identified as the useful many. The Pareto chart is based on the 80/20 rule; however, the team leaders need to understand that the rule is subject to variation, and the results must be carefully evaluated. This means that Choice *A* is incorrect. The Pareto chart only measures the frequencies of identified criteria such as the number of occurrences, patient complaints, and severity of the error, which means that Choice *B* is incorrect. The useful many are the areas that are performing well, so root cause analysis would not be appropriate for these areas. Therefore, Choice *D* is incorrect.

**103. B:** The Statistical Process Control (SPC) chart evaluates the variation in a project to identify the common cause and the special cause variants. Common cause variation is due to chance and will not affect the process outcomes. Special cause variants represent an error in the process that will negatively affect process outcomes. These variations must be identified and eliminated. This means that Choice *B* is the correct answer. The Pareto analysis identifies the frequency of a problem and the area that is responsible for that problem. The chart provides information according to the eighty-twenty rule rather than identifying the specific characteristics of process variation, which means that Choice *A* is incorrect.

Choice *C* is incorrect because FMEA analysis (failure mode and effects analysis) predicts possible errors and estimates the effects of those errors on the customer. Choice *D* is incorrect because the fishbone is used to assess cause and effect, not variation characteristics.

**104. D:** By definition, the $RC^2$ analysis includes an action plan that is not included in FMEA or SBAR, and the resulting data can be used to submit information to the Joint Commission. According to some authorities, the $RC^2$ measure is more comprehensive and therefore more reliable than the FMEA, which means that Choice *A* is incorrect. Choice *B* is incorrect because SBAR is a communication framework that does not include a remediation plan. The $RCA^2$ is used to report sentinel event data to the Joint Commission, which means that Choice *C* is incorrect.

**105. B:** Competitive benchmarking is a process that team leaders use to identify the characteristics of other successful organizations. The team leaders can then compare the KPIs for both organizations. However, the indicators are relative to several organizational characteristics (such as the geographic location, patient demographics, and university affiliations), so the comparisons must account for these individual differences. For example, the KPIs for a hospital in an urban setting in Alabama are different than the indicators for a community hospital in the "ski country" of Colorado. Competitive benchmarking does not rely on a single KPI, because one measure (e.g., hospital bed capacity) would not provide a comprehensive picture of any organization. This means that Choice *A* is incorrect. Hospitals in the same geographic location also can vary on several metrics that would invalidate the comparison. For instance, readmission rates for a hospital that serves a vulnerable population will not compare with readmission rates of a private-care hospital that provides excellent orthopedic care. This means that Choice *C* is incorrect. KPIs are sensitive to patient demographics, which means that Choice *D* is incorrect.

**106. D:** Generic benchmarking compares a general concept between two unrelated organizations. For instance, hospital team leaders could compare employee satisfaction rates with data from the United Autoworkers. Competitive benchmarking compares a similar process between two similar organizations, such as comparing Hospital A's readmission rates for patients with heart failure with Hospital B's rate. This means that Choice *A* is incorrect. Internal benchmarking is the comparison of an equivalent process in two different groups in the same organization. For instance, the number of sick days recorded for human resources and environmental services could be compared. This means that Choice *B* is incorrect. Functional benchmarking compares similar processes in different types of organizations. For instance, hospitals could compare performance appraisal procedures with a widget production company. This means that Choice *D* is incorrect.

**107. D:** The equation is frequently described as a "breakthrough equation" because it can identify cause and effect, evaluate performance, and reveal areas for potential improvement. An example in healthcare might be measuring the success of a process aimed at increasing the number of diabetic eye check visits in an outpatient clinic. The "Y" represents the number of visits that are scheduled. The "*f*" would be the number of emails sent via the patient portal, and the (*n*) would be the five-dollar e-coupon to the Widget store for scheduling the visit. This means that Choice *D* is the correct answer. The equation is commonly used in other process improvement models, so Choice *A* is incorrect. Choice *B* is incorrect because the model provides useful information for every step of the DMAIC process; for instance, in the "M" or measure step, the "*x*" can be used to identify significant factors or inputs that are required to obtain the desired outcomes. The scope of the equation goes beyond process improvement; therefore, Choice *C* is incorrect.

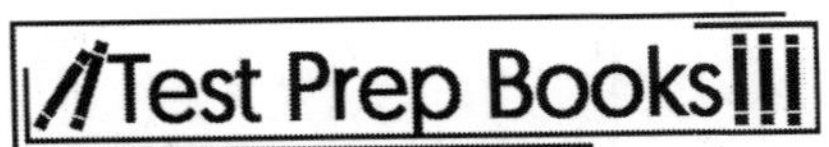

**108. D:** The Hospital Consumer Assessment of Healthcare Providers and Systems (HCAHPS) survey was developed to provide a standardized approach to the measurement of patient satisfaction in nineteen areas including pain management, provider communication, and discharge planning. Some providers have criticized the survey's use as a reimbursement metric because the results may not be consistently correlated with KPIs such as post-operative opioid therapy and, most importantly, clinical outcomes. Choice *A* is incorrect because the correlation between postoperative pain management is not always associated with increased patient satisfaction. As noted, researchers have expressed concerns about the lack of a consistent correlation between patient satisfaction and clinical outcomes. This means that Choice *B* is incorrect. The survey results affect CMS payments in all states regardless of Medicaid programs, which means that Choice *C* is incorrect.

**109. A:** The return on the investment (ROI) provides the "bottom line" indicator for the success of the Six Sigma initiative because it addresses the reason that the company exists, which means that Choice *A* is correct. The remaining choices all contribute to the success of the improvement plan; however, each measure is relevant to one area of process improvement rather than providing an all-inclusive view of the process. Choice *B* is incorrect because the identification of cause and effect looks at potential process errors rather than the success of the entire process. Choice *C* is incorrect because failure potential identifies possible errors and their impact on customer satisfaction. Pilot testing results are used to evaluate the initial use of the updated process in real-time, so Choice *D* is incorrect.

**110. A:** Groupthink occurs when the entire group becomes focused on a single idea or solution in the early stages of the brainstorming session. This tends to occur in groups with one or two strong voices who can quickly influence the remaining participants, thereby limiting the identification of additional good ideas. Experts encourage team leaders to plan for groupthink by requiring that all group members come to the session with three to five ideas on paper. The problem identified with groupthink is the limited number of ideas as opposed to the plausibility of the solutions, which means that Choice *B* is incorrect. The group members are appropriately engaged in the process, but they become focused on a single solution very early in the group process. This single solution may or may not be the best solution. This means that Choice *C* is incorrect. Capable leadership is required to avoid the development of groupthink and to maintain the integrity of the quality improvement efforts. Choice *D* is incorrect because groupthink does not affect the self-reliance of the group.

**111. B:** The team leader discusses key points in the Know How segment of the model. The talking object is passed among the team members who contribute individually to the discussion of the Key Points as noted in the meeting agenda. The Know What segment of the model addresses the steps required for an effective information huddle. Successful huddles occur when the agenda is followed, all individuals are prepared to participate, and the meetings are brief and conclude on time. The Know Why segment of the model provides the reasons for the key points. Choices *A* and *C* are incorrect because the key points are discussed in the Know How segment of the model. Choice *D* is incorrect because no segment is specifically identified as the introduction.

**112. D:** Choice *D* is correct because the team leader's most important function in the initial stage of Tuckman's model is the promotion of team interaction, which enhances communication at all levels. Reflecting on the group process occurs in the adjourning stage, so Choice *A* is incorrect. Conflicts occur in the storming stage, so Choice *B* is incorrect. Identifying the competence of individual team members occurs in the performing stage, so Choice *C* is incorrect.

**113. A:** The Science of Improvement identifies three types of healthcare improvement measures: outcome, process, and balancing measures. Outcome measures identify performance results. Process measures assess the effects of care on the patient, the organization, or the community. Balancing measures assess the possible impact of one improvement process on another measure. For example, if using the ventilator bundle protocol results in earlier extubation, will re-intubation rates increase? Choice *B* is incorrect because semi-annual testing is a process measure. The number of adverse drug reactions per quarter is an outcome measure, which means that Choice *C* is incorrect. Completion of on-time intentional rounding is a process measure, so Choice *D* is also incorrect.

**114. A:** The *analyze* step of the DMAIC framework involves comparing current data with the proposed outcome measure. For instance, if the proposed outcome measure states that one hundred percent of eligible clinic patients will receive flu shots by October 31, the analyze step will divide the actual number of patients who received flu shots by October 31 by one hundred (from the outcome measure). Choice *B* is incorrect because it is an outcome measure that is identified in the *define* step of the DMAIC process. Choice *C* is incorrect because tracking systems are addressed in the *improve* step of the model. Choice *D* is incorrect because applying a tracking protocol to an additional outcome measure would be addressed in the *control* step of the model.

**115. C:** Organizations that choose to accept the rules for the CMS Advanced Alternative Payment Model (APM) do assume additional financial risk; however, the organizations also receive greater financial incentives for meeting care outcomes. Smaller group practices most commonly choose the Merit-Based Incentive Payment System (MIPS), which is associated with less risk and lower incentives for value-based care. The use of EHR utilization is required for all organizations, which means that Choice *A* is incorrect.

Organizations that participate in the MIPS system receive less incentive money than the APM organizations, which means that Choice *B* is incorrect. All provider groups are eligible for at least one of the payment plans; however, the eligibility rules for single and group providers are based on the percentage of income received from Medicare Part B or the percentage of Medicare patients cared for by the provider or group of providers. For example, under the 2020 rules, to become a qualifying participant in the APM model, a group of providers would need to either receive 50 percent of all Medicare Part B reimbursement as a member of that group or each group member would need to care for 35 percent of all Medicare reimbursed patient care in the group. This means that Choice *D* is incorrect.

**116. C:** The SHARE model (Seek, Help, Assess, Reach, Evaluate) is focused on facilitating the patient's ability to make informed care decisions that are consistent with evidence-based practice and their values. The process involves providing the patient with the best treatment options, exploring the patient's preferences and values, helping the patient to make a decision, and evaluating the effects of that decision. The Assess step of the model addresses the patient's personal values rather than their disease process, which means that Choices *A* and *B* are incorrect. The financial impact of the patient's diagnosis will influence the identification of the treatment plan in the Help step; however, the Assess step is focused on the patient's values. This means that Choice *D* is also incorrect.

**117. A:** The correct choice is the direct manager because that person is in the best position to identify individuals with the necessary skills needed for a successful team member. Choice *B* is incorrect because although peer evaluation may reflect some of the criteria for team membership, the direct manager is better prepared to evaluate all critical performance criteria. Choice *C* is incorrect because the senior manager receives information about individual performance from the direct manager. A self-evaluation

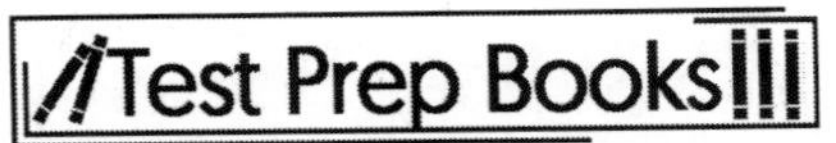

is an important tool in performance assessment; however, it may or may not coincide with the company requirements for a given position, so Choice *D* is incorrect.

**118. B:** The focus of the SHARE model is the patient's experience with decision-making and the outcomes of those decisions. Cost of care is not a specific outcome. Choices *A, C,* and *D* are intended outcomes for the model, which means they are incorrect.

**119. B:** The AI natural language processing (NLP) model is currently being used to make narrative EHR data intelligible for data capture. Predictive analytical models use time-sequenced data for the EHR to suggest the patient's prognosis. These models do not rely on NLP, which means that Choice *A* is incorrect. The care decision algorithms are added to the EHR databases and are triggered by patient data; however, the systems do not depend on NLP, so Choice *C* is incorrect. Other forms of AI, rather than NLP, are also responsible for the currently limited application of AI to diagnostic radiology, which means that Choice *D* is incorrect.

**120. D:** Force field analysis is one form of process assessment that identifies all factors that favor the success of the proposed innovation as compared to all factors that are potential barriers to the successful implementation of the new process. This exercise is seen as an important first step assessment, so that means that Choice *D* is correct. The remaining choices are incorrect because they represent individual assessments that are not related to the force field analysis.

**121. D:** The CAHPS output is patient satisfaction information related to individual insurance plans and organizations that can be used by patients to assess the available healthcare resources. The HEDIS databases can be used for competitive benchmarking, organizational data analytics, and research. Reporting for the HEDIS databases is not based on patient input, which means that Choice *A* is incorrect. Core measures reporting is completed by hospitals and providers to document value-based care. Consumer input is not the focus of these measures, so Choice *B* is incorrect. The AHIP reports might be used by consumers; however, the intent was to standardize reporting measures used by insurance plans. This means that Choice *C* is incorrect.

**122. D:** Medicare patients may not have access to the new biosimilar and generic drugs because Part D plans have been slow to add the drugs to plan formularies. In addition, the United States Inspector General found that even when the drug was in the plan formulary, the placement of the drug in the "tiered" framework also limited patient access. Choice *A* is incorrect because there are biosimilar drugs for hypertension and many other common illnesses. There is no evidence that patients are reluctant to take these drugs; patients are familiar with the concept of generic drugs, which has contributed to their acceptance of biosimilar drugs, which means that Choice *B* is incorrect. Interchangeability is the degree to which the "similar" drug is equivalent to the action of the original drug concerning chemical purity and patient response. All biosimilar drugs must meet the Food and Drug Administration (FDA) interchangeability standard, which means that Choice *C* is incorrect.

**123. B:** Choice *B* is correct because the work package is used to divide the larger project into workable steps toward completion of the project, which then forms the basis for project evaluation. Choice *A* is incorrect because the work package is not directly associated with production costs. Choice *C* is incorrect because inventory control is not a component of the work package criteria. Choice *D* is incorrect because the work package is not related to performance assessment.

**124. B:** The Hospital Value-Based Purchasing Program was initiated to change the way hospitals are paid for caring for patients covered by Medicare. Instead of the fee-for-service model, the Hospital Value-Based Purchasing Program reimburses hospitals based on patient-care outcomes. Currently, scores for Clinical Outcomes, Community and Person Engagement, Safety, and Cost Reduction are equally weighted at 25 percent of the total score. Under this program, there are no additional incentives for individual diseases. The program applies to all patient care reimbursed by Medicare, which means that Choice *A* is incorrect. As noted, the clinical outcomes score is one of four measures included in the program, so Choice *C* is incorrect. Only acute-care hospitals, rather than outpatient or ambulatory care providers, are eligible for this reimbursement program. That means that Choice *D* is incorrect.

**125. B:** Next-generation data management systems require that EHR data is retrievable as intelligible information consistent with structured terminologies. The controlled medical library of structured terminologies will consist of prescribed EHR documentation entries that will facilitate communication among systems and support data management requirements. Narrative EHR data is not well understood electronically because of the free-form nature of the information, which means that all providers must use the alternative prescribed terminology to document care. This deficit affects the entire system, because organizations are not able to capture accurate data for required activities such as outcomes reporting or claims processing. Medical terminologies require software integration rather than hardware considerations, which means that Choice *A* is incorrect. The use of the prescribed language is related to communication and data retrieval rather than security, which means that Choice *C* is incorrect. The immediate staff learning needs will increase substantially because all forms of data entry will be affected by the implementation of the structured data entry and formatting. This means that Choice *D* is incorrect.

# Index

Dear CPHQ Test Taker,

We would like to start by thanking you for purchasing this study guide for your CPHQ exam. We hope that we exceeded your expectations.

Our goal in creating this study guide was to cover all of the topics that you will see on the test. We also strove to make our practice questions as similar as possible to what you will encounter on test day. With that being said, if you found something that you feel was not up to your standards, please send us an email and let us know.

We have study guides in a wide variety of fields. If you're interested in one, try searching for it on Amazon or send us an email.

Thanks Again and Happy Testing!
Product Development Team
info@studyguideteam.com

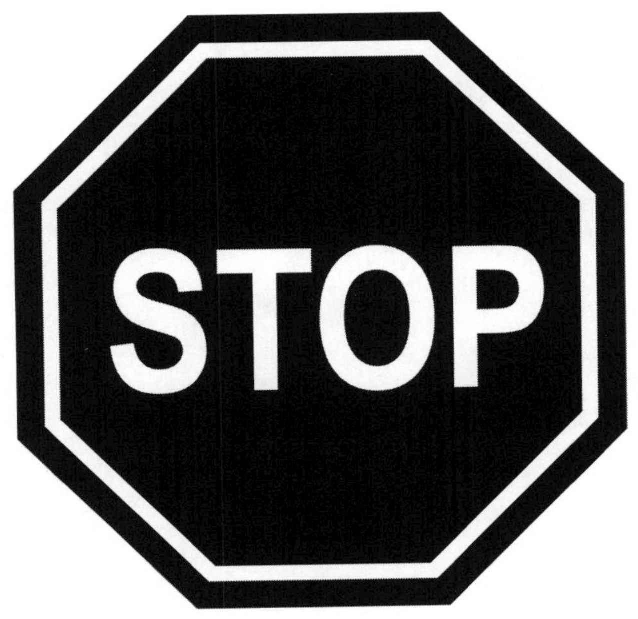


# FREE Test Taking Tips Video/DVD Offer

To better serve you, we created videos covering test taking tips that we want to give you for FREE. **These videos cover world-class tips that will help you succeed on your test.**

We just ask that you send us feedback about this product. Please let us know what you thought about it—whether good, bad, or indifferent.

To get your **FREE videos**, you can use the QR code below or email freevideos@studyguideteam.com with "Free Videos" in the subject line and the following information in the body of the email:

a. The title of your product

b. Your product rating on a scale of 1-5, with 5 being the highest

c. Your feedback about the product

If you have any questions or concerns, please don't hesitate to contact us at info@studyguideteam.com.

Thank you!

Made in the USA
Coppell, TX
02 May 2023